IRISH FOLK MEDICINE

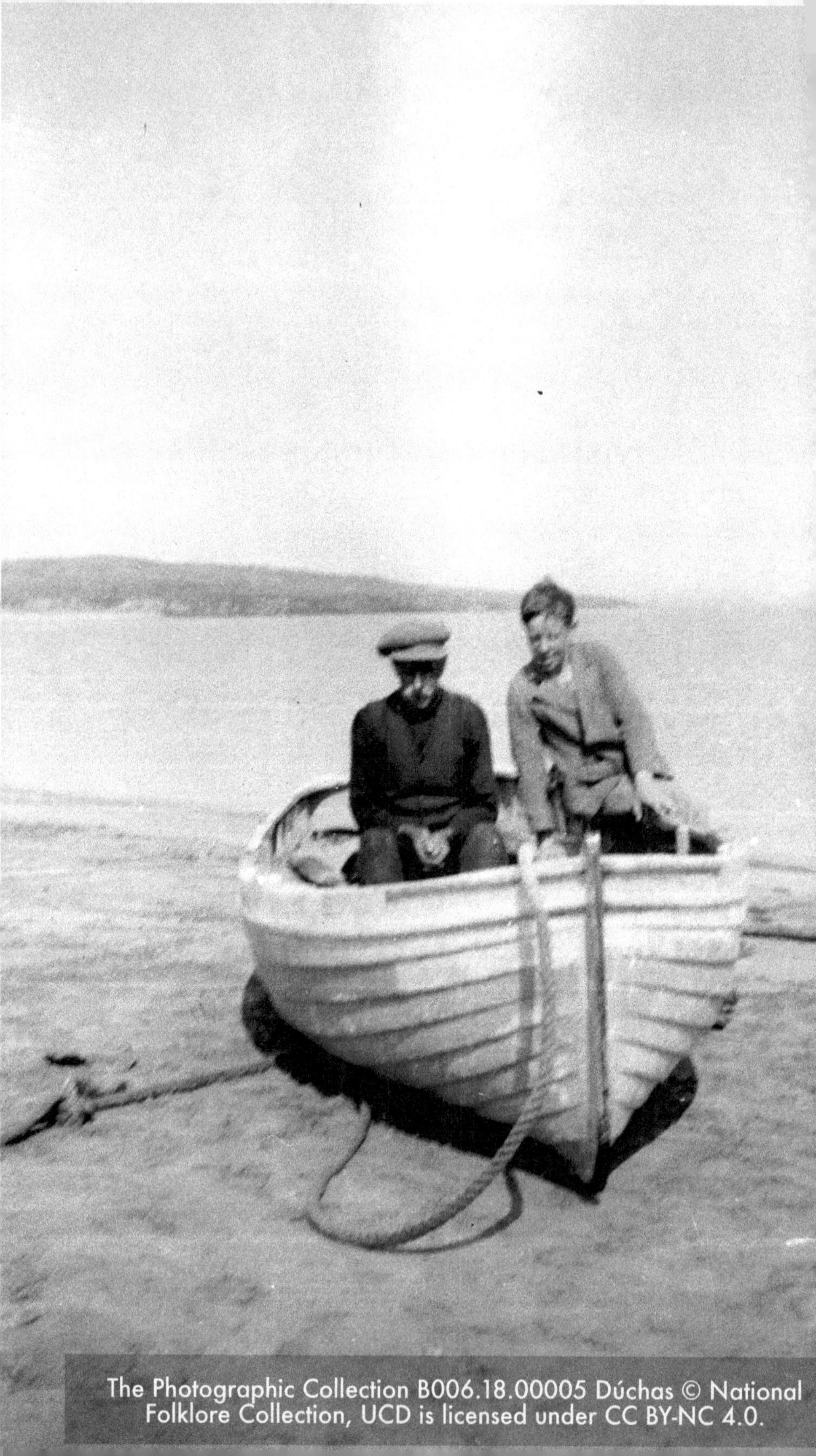

IRISH FOLK MEDICINE

Herbal Remedies from the Irish Schools Collection

Fiona Forde

AEON

First published in 2026 by
Aeon Books

British Library Cataloguing in Publication Data

A C.I.P. for this book is available from the British Library

ISBN-13: 978-1-80152-249-6

Typeset by Alice Rathbone

www.aeonbooks.co.uk

Disclaimer:
Every effort has been made to ensure that the information in the book is accurate. The information in this book may not be applicable in each individual case so it is advised that professional medical advice is obtained for specific health matters and before changing any medication or dosage. The author accepts no legal responsibility for any personal injury or other damage or loss arising from the use of the information in this book. Errors may have crept in, due diligence and repeated fact-checking are still fallible. If you find any errors please contact the author or publisher so any further editions can be corrected.

CONTENTS

25. 5.

Cures.

There are not as many cu[res]
now as there were long ago.
My Grandmother told me a f[ew]
Nettles are very good to eat [dur-]
ing the month of March, an[d]
it is said that you should [boil]
them and eat them three ti[mes]
during the month. and the
person that does this will
not get any disease during
the year.
The roots of docket leaves b[oil-]
-ed in milk are said to cu[re]
a sick stomack.
Garlic boiled in milk is g[ood]
for a cold. and to put so[me]
into your shoes would cu[re]
rheumatism.

Bridgie Ryan.
Menlough. G. S.

Told by. Mrs Ryan. age 89
Ballinamona

There are not as many cures now as there were long ago.

My Grandmother told me a few.

(1) Nettles are very good to eat during the month of March, and it is said that you should boil them and eat them three times during the month, and the person that does this will not get any disease during the year.

(2) The roots of docket leaves boiled in milk are used to cure a sick stomach.

(3) Garlic boiled in milk is good for a cold, and to put some into your shoes would cure rheumatism.

INTRODUCTION

The Irish Folklore Commission

Séamus Ó Duilearga founded *An Cumann le Béaloideas Éireann* (The Folklore of Ireland Society) and its journal *Béaloideas* in 1927. The Irish Government then established the *Institiúid Bhéaloideas Éireann* (The Irish Folk Institute) in 1930, to be headed by Ó Duilearga, with other board members of An Cumann recruited alongside (Almqvist, 1977–79: 9).

The Irish Folklore Commission was set up in 1935 by the Irish government to study and collect information on the folklore and traditions of Ireland when a larger organisation that was better equipped was felt to be needed. Ó Duilearga was appointed honorary director of the Commission, and led its effort (Almqvist, 1977–79: 22; Briody, 2007: 2, 232). The Commission was responsible for the collection and preservation of Irish folk tradition of all forms, with the additional tasks of cataloguing the material under classification, their study and exposition (Almqvist, 1977–79: 9).

The Commission focused on Ireland's diverse populations. The Commission was closely involved with locals, especially Irish-speaking districts. They distributed questionnaires and used media outlets to inform the general public of the Commission.

With greater recognition, Ó Duilearga's vision for the Commission grew, and around the 1950s many scholars were participating by contributing to collections and research (Briody, 2007: 21).

The Commission continued its work by that name until 1971 when it was superseded by the Department of Irish Folklore in the University College, Dublin (Almqvist, 1977–79: 21). The department has since served as a repository of the data collected, including the Irish Folklore Collection, which later became the National Folklore Collection, at the UCD Delargy Centre for Irish Folklore and the National Folklore Collection (Briody, 2007: 490).

The Schools' Collection

Among the Irish Folklore Commission's collections are written interviews recorded between 1937 and 1939. Known collectively as *The Schools' Collection,* these interviews were conducted by more than 50,000 schoolchildren from all primary schools in the South of Ireland.

From 1937 to 1939, the students collected some 740,000 pages of folklore and local tradition (288,000 pages in the students' original exercise books and 451,000 pages in bound volumes).

The Department of Education and the Irish National Teachers' Association were key partners in this collection programme.

The 1,128 volumes include written accounts of daily life as well as regional folklore and stories as told by the interviewees (*The Dúchas Project. Retrieved 22 September 2018).*

The project involved the children gathering folklore in their local communities. In several instances, the programme was extended until 1939 from its intended 1937–38 term.

This was instigated by Sean Ó Súilleabháin and Séamus Ó Duilearga, who publicised the scheme and explained to teachers what folklore was and how to properly collect it (Briody, 2007: 268–9). They met with principal teachers, who then explained to the children how to collect the folklore for the collection. They received a grant from the Rockefeller Foundation of $500. From September to June, each week the teacher would choose a heading and read out the questions, and the children would copy it down and question their family members and neighbours. In June 1939, Ó Duilearga stated in his annual report that there were collectively 375,660 pages of books from the schools (Briody, 2007: 267).

Oral history, trades and crafts, games and pastimes, proverbs and riddles, topography, folktales and legends, and more are all covered in the Collection. This information was gathered by the children from their parents, grandparents and neighbours.

The Collection consists of 1,128 bound and numbered volumes. A further collection of approximately 40,000 of the children's original copybooks is held by the National Folklore Commission.

Dúchas Project

The Dúchas Project is an online crowdsourcing effort to digitize and transcribe the National Folklore Collection in order to make it accessible and searchable worldwide. Based online, the project includes (1) both digitised and transcribed volumes of the collection; (2) a search feature to find people, topics and places mentioned in the collections; (3) an index of Irish surnames, and (4) numerous historical photographs (*www.duchas.ie/en.. Retrieved 22 September 2018*).

Transcriptions of the Collection are crowdsourced from around the world, and volunteers transcribe pages from the journal, allowing each page transcribed to become searchable from within the page itself and via internet search databases.

The material is taken directly from Dúchas.ie without further interpretation or editing.

What we can learn from our ancestors

The Schools' Collection records, among other things, show how the local communities in Ireland were using herbal remedies up to 1939. While many of the herbs used and the use to which they were put to is unsurprising, what is incredible is the lesser known uses of those herbs that were well known and understood by these local communities. In a time before the internet or access to written records about these herbs, it is truly fascinating to compare the easy and natural relationship these communities had with the plants and how the cohesiveness of that local plant and human relationship led to an understanding of the various remedies the plants could offer. For many of us living in this information-soaked age with an abundance of research papers, books and findings, it is truly humbling to appreciate how simply living with and treating these plants with the respect they deserve afforded these communities so much in terms of medicine. The study of the Schools' Collection really teaches us about:

- A sense of community
- Utilising local herbs
- Wisdom shared through generations

The Photographic Collection

Members of the Irish Folklore Commission (1935–70) and its successors, including staff of the National Folklore Collection, took the majority of the 80,000 images in the National Folklore Collection's photographic collection. Livelihoods, crafts, trade, transportation, the sea, education, religious practice, cuisine, clothes, festivals and rites of passage, pastimes, sports, singers, storytellers and vernacular homes are among the themes.

How to approach this book

This book is an appreciation of how community knowledge, folk practice and modern herbalism interweave. It references various historical Irish herbal folk cures, built around material from the Schools' Collection and the National Folklore Collection, and paired with contemporary herbal commentary and recipes.

Overall layout

- The opening sections introduce the Irish Folklore Commission, the Schools' Collection and the Dúchas digital project, explaining who collected the material, how it was gathered, and how it is now preserved and accessed.

- The school children's accounts from the Schools' Collection are reproduced directly from the transcriptions on dúchas.ie, without further editing, and point the reader back to the original manuscripts and digitised volumes.

Plant-by-plant chapters

- The main body of the book is organised plant by plant (for example carrageen moss, chamomile, comfrey, dandelion, ivy, mugwort, yarrow and others), each with a short identification section.

Photos, graphics and references

- Throughout, there are referenced photos from the National Folklore Collection's Photographic Collection, which visually ground the text in rural Irish life.

Editorial Note

Accounts from the Schools' Collection have been reproduced in this book from the transcribed material available on dúchas.ie, with permission from the National Folklore Collection, UCD. The accounts have been reproduced directly, without further editing. The original manuscripts can be found in the National Folklore Collection and their digitised counterparts can be found on dúchas.ie.

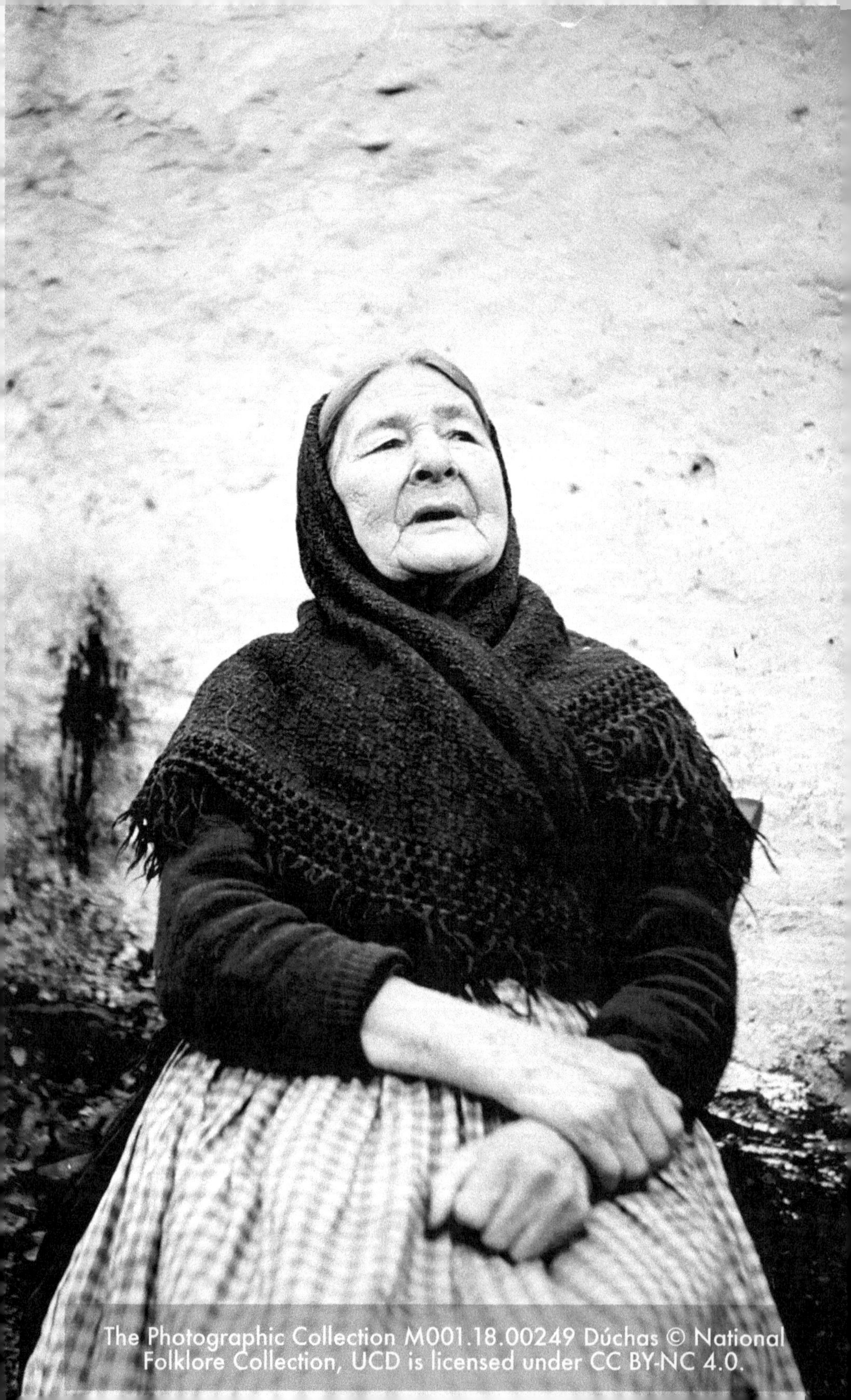

BARBERRY

Berberis vulgaris (syn. B. aetnensis, B. boisseri, B. orientalis)

The School's Collection, Volume 0496, Page 0058

Long ago, when doctors were not so numerous, people relied more on the local cures. Herbs were used mostly by everybody, to cure their diseases. Yarrow and celery seed, are great cure for rheumatism, and the old people rely on them yet, and it is still used.

A great for "thrush" is for a child born after its fathers death to breathe into the sick childs mouth.

The cure for the jaundice is to get the bark of the barberry tree, and to boil it in milk, and to drink the milk. The dock leaf is a great cure for a nettle burn

The School's Collection, Volume 0495, Page 0247

1. A maried woman's ring would cure a sty by blessing yourself with it.

2. Pepper is used for curing a toothache.
3. The bark of the Barberry tree cures the Jaundice.
4. Dandeline cures the liver complaint.
5. The snails gathered on the due on the morning cures consumption.
6. The food left behind after a ferret is supposed to be able to cure the chin-cough.

The School's Collection, Volume 0496, Page 0058

The cure for the jaundice is to get the bark of the barberry tree, and to boil it in milk, and to drink the milk. The dock leaf is a great cure for a nettle burn.

The School's Collection, Volume 0495, Page 0247

The bark of the Barberry tree cures the Jaundice.

The reference to jaundice is consistent with the traditional use of barberry as a remedy for correcting liver function and encouraging bile flow, in particular when gallstones or gallbladder inflammation are present, and when jaundice results from liver congestion. In those who are weak or incapacitated, it helps strengthen and cleanse the system as a bitter tonic with mild laxative effects (Hoffmann, 2003).

In *The Complete Herbal*, originally published in 1653, Culpeper (1995) recommends the daily consumption of barberry decoction, which was believed to clear the body of choleric humours and free it from choler, yellow jaundice, scabs, itch, skin conditions, fevers, dysentery, and other ailments associated with hot-temperedness (Culpeper, 1653/1995).

Traditionally, different parts of barberry were used in cases of an enlarged liver or spleen, eye sores, toothache, asthma, dry skin, ulcers, and jaundice (Rahimi-Madiseh et al., 2017).

Barberry recipes

Wound wash

Barberry and yarrow are helpful wound herbs as they are antimicrobial and vulnerary.

1 tbsp (0.5 fl oz) yarrow (*Achillea millefolium*) aerial parts tincture

1½ tsp calendula (*Calendula officinalis*) flower tincture

1½ tsp barberry (*Berberis spp.)* root tincture

1. Combine tinctures in a 1-ounce glass dropper bottle.
2. Shake well.
3. Label, and store in a cool, dark place.
4. To use, pour 1–2 droppersful on minor wounds.

Safety consideration

Avoid during pregnancy.

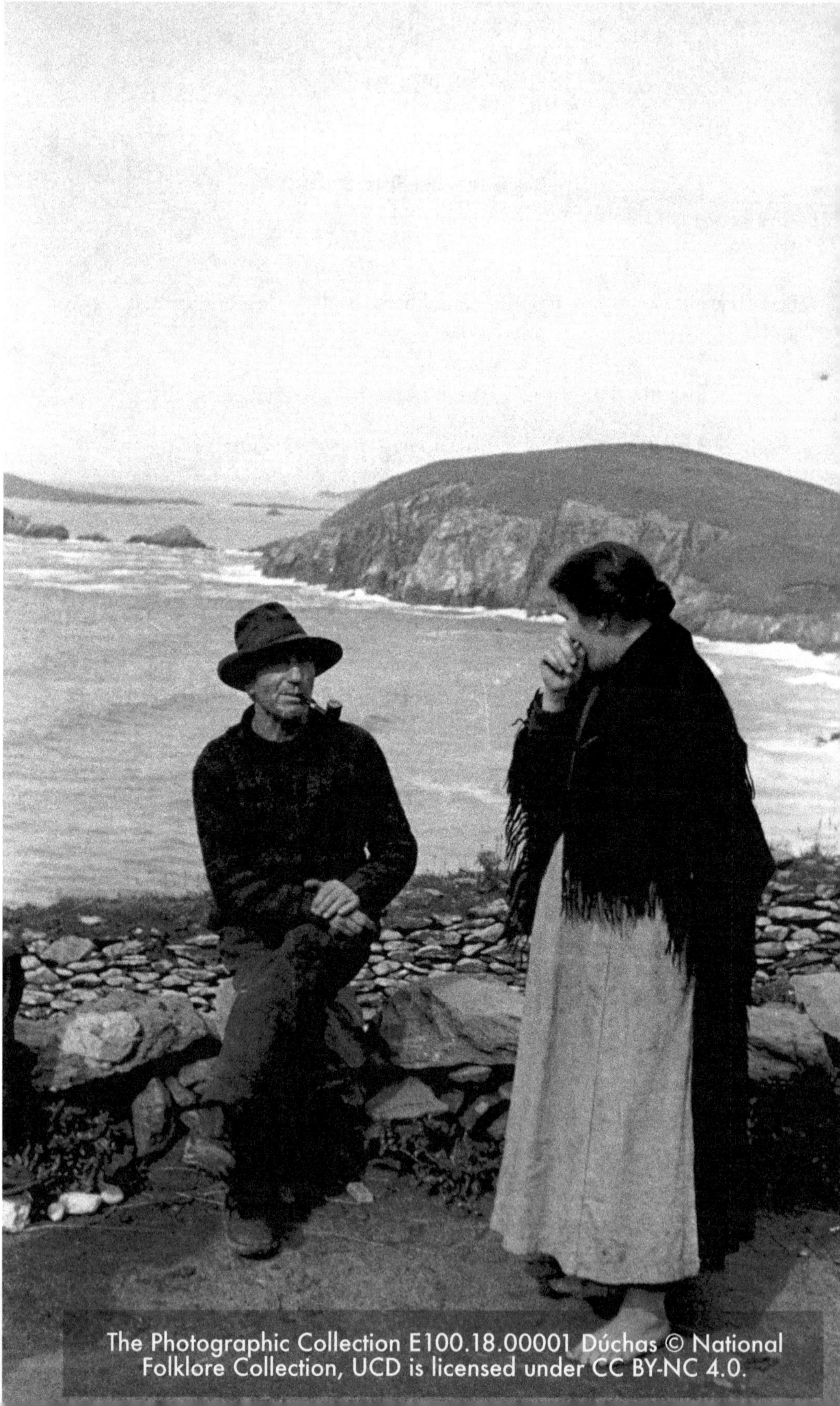

CARRAGEEN MOSS (IRISH MOSS)

Chondrus crispus

The School's Collection, Volume 0053, Page 0120

For the yellow-jaundice. Carrigeen moss is used for coughs and is got on the sea shore. Ivy leaf is great for burns Briar leaves are used for scalds. A dogleaf is a cure for burns of nettles People say that the wild tea cures cancer It grows in the ditches. Groundsel is used for feeding birds. Some people boil nettles and eat them. There was a herb called gladam. First they would pound the gladam and put it to your neck and leave it twenty four hours on. They say it always cured the mumps.

There is another herb called anlóg. It scatters and destroys crops. There is an old saying about the preasac buidhe "one year's growing means seven years' weeding". Garlic is a cure for bad rash on the face.

Coughs

The School's Collection, Volume 0053, Page 0120

Carrigeen moss is used for coughs and is got on the sea shore.

Since Carrageen moss was traditionally used to cure respiratory illnesses, including bronchitis, annoying coughs, and several other lung issues, the aforementioned use of the moss is not particularly surprising.

Carrageen moss – other uses

Carrageen moss is also often used for digestive disorders like gastritis and duodenal and stomach ulcers that call for a demulcent. It is beneficial for inflammations of the urinary system owing to its soothing properties. Additionally, it has been incorporated into maintenance diets for diabetics. Historically, carrageen was used to aid in the recovery from debilitating illness. After a serious illness, herbs like Irish moss and other nutritive tonics can help with recovery.

Irish moss was recommended by King in 1898 as a demulcent for chronic airway disorders, rickets, chronic diarrhoea and dysentery, and kidney and bladder irritation. Irish moss may impair absorption of drugs (Hoffmann, 2003).

Carrageen moss recipes

Carrageen moss pudding

8g cleaned, dried carrageen moss (*Chondrus crispus*)

800ml full-fat milk

100ml cream

1 tbsp caster sugar

1 vanilla pod or ½ tsp pure vanilla extract

1 free range egg

1. Soak the carrageen in cold water for 10 minutes or until it has swelled and increased in size. Drain.

2. Put the carrageen moss, milk, and vanilla pod (if using) in a saucepan. Bring to a boil, then cover and simmer gently for 20 minutes.

3. Separate the egg, place the yolk in a bowl and whisk in the sugar and, if using, vanilla essence.

4. Pour the milk and carrageen moss mixture through a strainer into the egg yolk mixture and add the cream while swirling constantly.

5. Cover with clingfilm and chill until ready to serve.

Safety consideration

May impair absorption of drugs (Hoffmann, 2003).

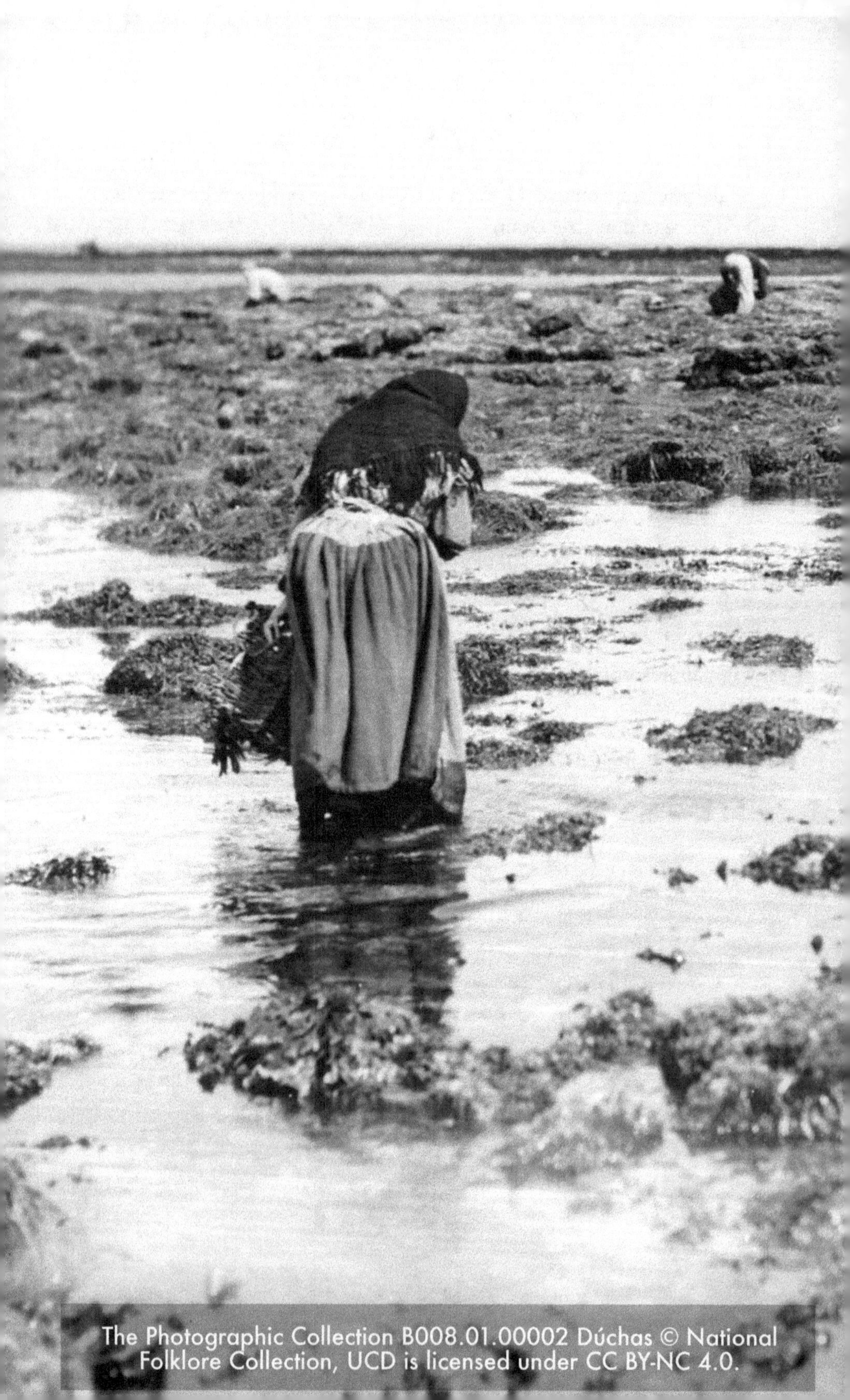

CHAMOMILE

Matricaria chamomilla

The School's Collection, Volume 0050, Page 0469

The most harmful weed growing on the farm at home is the yellow dock because they spread rapidly and impoverish the land. The thistle is the plant most common that grows on good land.
The following are the herbs found on our farm and their cures. Chamomile for nervousness and debility. Dandelion a laxative and a tonic. Clover is used for colds, etc. Comfrey fine medicine for chest complaints also poultices. Red Dock an excellent blood purifier.

The School's Collection, 0050, Pages 0458–0461

Tradition tell us that the people of older times were much healthier than the people are nowadays. The only cure they had for any illness they might have were herbs.
The sowed those herbs in gardens, the same as we would sow vegetables now, but the bog-onion grew in bogs, or the banks of some rivers, or streams.

Swelling

The School's Collection, Volume 0057, Page 0124

Chamomile Flowers. Boil flowers and use water for swellings of the face in cases of abscesses, bad teeth, etc.

Chamomile has been used to soothe colds, minor ulcers and inflammations of the mouth and throat, and topically applied to ease irritations and minor inflammations of the skin, such as sunburn and superficial wounds (European Medicines Agency, 2015).

Earaches

The School's Collection, Volume 0050, Page 0460

Camomile flowers are boiled and applied for poultices for the ear. They are found to be the best cure going.

The anti-inflammatory qualities of chamomile may help to explain this reference. According to Chevallier (2007), chamomile is an anti-inflammatory herb that can be applied topically to skin irritations such as rashes, abrasions, and insect bites and stings. The German Commission E monographs infer that chamomile can be applied topically to skin inflammations and bacterial skin conditions (Blumenthal, 1998). In the past, chamomile has been used as a vulnerary to assist with healing wounds (Srivastava et al., 2010). The beneficial effects of chamomile on the skin have been well documented (Merfort et al., 1994).

Chamomile recipes

Calming chamomile cream

A soothing cream for skin inflammation, rosacea-prone or sensitive skin and hives.

⅓ cup (2.7 fl oz) chamomile (*Matricaria chamomilla*) flower-infused jojoba oil

2½ tbsp (1.25 fl oz) coconut oil

2 tbsp beeswax

½ tsp vitamin E oil

⅓ cup (2.7 fl oz) well-strained liquorice (*Glycyrrhiza glabra*) root decoction

2½ tbsp (1.25 fl oz) aloe (Aloe vera) leaf gel

4–5 drops chamomile (*Matricaria chamomilla*) flower essential oil (optional)

Natural preservative (optional)

1. Make a decoction using 4 tbsp liquorice root to 1 cup water, simmering for 20–30 minutes.
2. Let cool, then strain. Add aloe gel.
3. Put the coconut oil, beeswax and chamomile-infused oil in a double boiler over low heat (or place a glass bowl over a saucepan of simmering water) until the coconut oil and beeswax have melted. Blend by stirring.
4. Remove from heat and transfer to a blender or a bowl (if using immersion blender) to cool.
5. Allow oil mixture to cool to room temperature
6. Slowly add liquorice decoction mixture to oil mixture while blending on a low-medium setting. Mixture will begin to emulsify and become creamy.
7. Avoid over-mixing. The cream will set up as it cools. Add essential oils and stir to combine.

8. Pour cream into sterilised glass jars, label, and store in the refrigerator for 1–2 weeks

Chamomile scrub

Sea salt or sugar

Olive oil, or another oil of choice

Chamomile (*Matricaria chamomilla*) flower

1. Fill a container with sea salt or sugar and herbs, leaving room for oil.
2. Pour the oil over the contents just until saturated.
3. Add the ground herbs.

Calming and soothing skin lotion

7 drops chamomile (*Matricaria chamomilla*) essential oil

5 drops calendula (*Calendula officinalis*) essential oil

30ml jojoba oil

1. Mix essential oils and jojoba oil together.
2. Cover and shake well to combine.
3. Label, and store in a cool, dark place.

Digestive bitters

Bitters are used to support digestion through the action of the bitter taste, which stimulates digestive secretions.

2 tbsp dandelion (*Taraxacum officinale*) root

2 tbsp chamomile (*Matricaria chamomilla*) flower

2 tbsp orange (*Citrus* spp.) peel

1 tbsp burdock (*Arctium lappa*) root

1 cup vodka or brandy

1. Place herbs in a clean, dry glass jar, and completely cover them with alcohol.
2. Place parchment paper over the jar, then cover it with a lid, and label.
3. Put the jar somewhere dry and cool and let it macerate for four weeks.
4. When time is up, strain the herbs using a fine-mesh sieve with layered cheesecloth. Compost the herbs and reserve the liquid.
5. Place the liquid in glass dropper bottles, and label.
6. Take 3–5 drops directly on the tongue 15 minutes before meals to stimulate digestion.

Safety considerations

Chamomile may cause allergic reactions in people sensitive to plants in the Asteraceae family. However, such reactions are extremely rare (Hoffmann, 2003).

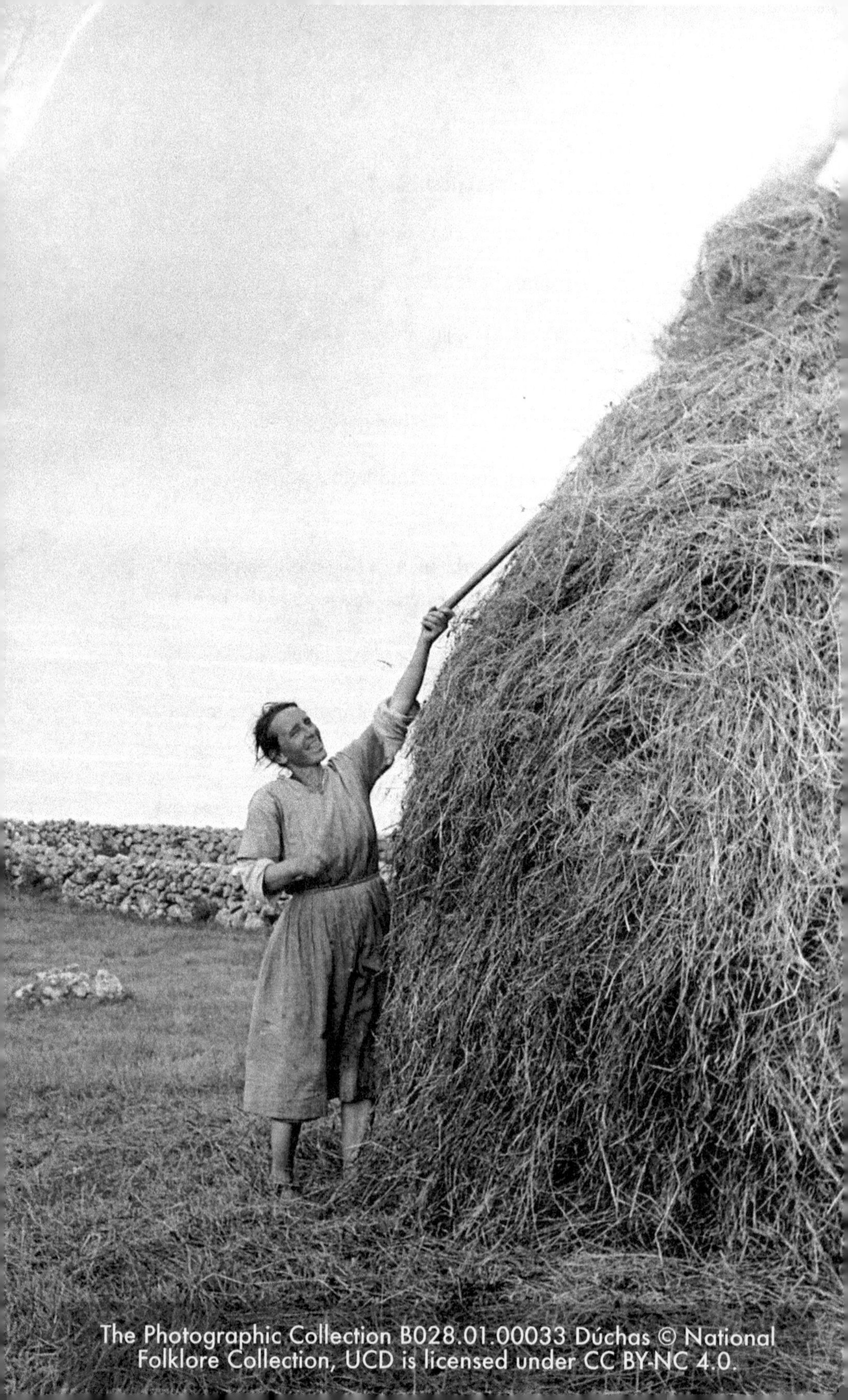

CHICKWEED / CHICKENWEED

Stellaria media

The Schools' Collection, Volume 0022, Page 0402

The herbs that grow in good land are farabán, chicken weed thistles, tansy and the daisy; In bad land dock leaves, nettles. The tansy is good for worms in horses. The nettles are good for rheumatism. The dock leaves are a cure for a burn from the nettle. There is a cure in the chicken weed for a running sore. The way the nettles are used to cure rheumatism is to boil them and drink the juice. The way the chicken weed is used for a sore is heat it in a pan and hit together and then leave it on the sore. The name of small tree that grows in the bog is the 'Reileog' and it never grew big because with that timber the cross was made on which Our Lord was crucified.

Swellings or sprains

The Schools' Collection, Volume 0004, Page 0332

Then there is the chicken-weed which is used to put down swellings or sprains.

Sores

The Schools' Collection, Volume 0022, Page 0402

There is a cure in the chicken weed for a running sore... The way the chicken weed is used for a sore is heat it in a pan and hit together and then leave it on the sore.

Chilblains

The Schools' Collection, Volume 0050, Page 0460

The chicken-weed grows, spread along the ground like moss. It is pounded also and found to be a good cure for chilblains.

Chickweed is an extremely lubricating herb with demulcent and emollient actions. It lubricates dry and irritated parts of the body both in the joints and topically on the skin. It is used to help moisten, cool and soothe irritation and inflammation throughout the body. Because of its lubricating qualities, people who eat it regularly often report a reduction in arthritis and rheumatic pain when consistently eating chickweed (Hoffmann, 2003).

Chickweed's moisturising and anti-inflammatory qualities make it a popular treatment for psoriasis, eczema and dry, itchy skin. Chickweed is often used as a salve or poultice, occasionally in combination with other calming and anti-inflammatory plants such as aloe (*Aloe vera*), calendula (*Calendula officinalis*), chamomile (*Matricaria chamomilla*), and plantain (*Plantago* spp.) (Klenner et al., 2015).

Chickweed can be consumed internally as a tea or meal for those with psoriasis and eczema. Preparations made from chickweed may also aid with various inflamed conditions such as wounds, rashes, burns and contact dermatitis (Wood, 2008).

Chickweed is a major herb for skin irritations, eye inflammation and kidney disorders. It is a mild diuretic and is indicated for water retention. It is an excellent poultice herb and is often found in salve formulas because of its soothing effects for the skin.

For cuts, bruises, burns, bites, and other skin irritation and inflammation, fresh, crushed chickweed leaves can be applied as a poultice (Blair, 2014). As a vulnerary herb, chickweed's cooling properties help to lessen the heat and inflammation of wounded tissues.

Chickweed is commonly used as an external remedy for cuts, wounds and, especially, itching and irritation. It may be used with benefit to treat eczema or psoriasis associated with this sort of irritation (Hoffmann, 2003).

Chickweed – other uses

Chickweed has a reputation as a remedy for rheumatism when used internally (Hoffmann, 2003). In the book *Physio-Medical Therapeutics, Materia Medica and Pharmacology* (Lyle, 1897), the author indicates chickweed for issues such as anaemia and rheumatism, stating that the herb stimulates circulation and mucous membranes, and improves appetite and digestion.

Chickweed is said to help balance the waters of the body by removing water from the kidneys and lymphatic congestion (Wood, 2008). It supports the kidneys and maintains the proper balance of water in the body by eliminating excess and keeping what is required. The passage and removal of toxins from the body via these organs and systems are supported by chickweed.

Herbalist Katrina Blair (2014) employs chickweed for removing congestion and infection from the body (p. 131). Chickweed's saponins aid in the assimilation and elimination of cysts and lumps as well as the dissolution of excesses in the body, including mucus, bacteria, undigested proteins and fat cells (Blair, 2014).

Irish Folk Medicine

The fresh tender greens are delicious in salads and are also nice juiced or blended in the blender with pineapple juice. Chickweed is a good source of nutrients and contains, among other nutrients, calcium, potassium and iron (Gladstar, 2012).

Chickweed recipes

Preparations and dosage

Chickweed is best taken fresh or as a water extract. In order to create an infusion, combine two teaspoons of the dried herb with one cup of boiling water and let it sit for five minutes. You can have this three times a day. Alternatively, you can put a handful of fresh chickweed and some pineapple juice in a blender and blend into a drink . A strong infusion of fresh plants can be added to bathwater to reduce itching (Hoffmann, 2003).

Diaper rash ointment

[Adapted from *Medical Herbalism* by David Hoffmann (2003)]

These herbs help to nourish and soothe the skin while protecting it from harmful bacteria and other pathogens. Comfrey (*Symphytum officinale*) leaf stimulates the growth of new tissue cells, and goldenseal (*Hydrastis canadensis*) root powder is a topical antimicrobial.

Apply ointment to diaper area after changing.

1 tablespoon chickweed (*Stellaria media*) leaf

1 tablespoon marshmallow (*Althaea officinalis*) root

1 tablespoon 2g (0.07 oz) comfrey (*Symphytum officinale*) root

1/8 teaspoon goldenseal (*Hydrastis canadensis*) powder

240 ml (8 fl oz) sweet almond oil

40g (1.4 oz) beeswax

1. Place sweet almond oil in a crock pot or double boiler with the herbs.
2. Steep on very low heat for 4–8 hours, being careful not to let herbs scorch or burn.
3. Strain mixture through cheesecloth and return to crock pot/double boiler.
4. Add the wax and allow it to melt.
5. After wax is melted, mix with a sterilised metal spoon and pour into a glass jar with a tight-fitting lid.
6. Label and place in fridge until mixture solidifies.
7. Store away from heat near infant's changing area.

Liver support soup

[Adapted from Rosemary Gladstar's *The Science and Art of Herbalism* course]

2 tbsp extra virgin olive oil

1 onion, chopped

3 garlic (*Allium sativum*) cloves, minced

2 inch piece fresh ginger (*Zingiber officinale*) rhizome, peeled and finely chopped

4 cups vegetable or chicken broth

1–2 fresh burdock (*Arctium lappa*) roots, chopped

2 carrots, sliced

⅓ cup red clover (*Trifolium pratense*) flower

1 bunch kale, finely chopped

2 parsnips, sliced

1 cup cabbage, finely shredded

1 handful fresh nettle (*Urtica dioica*) leaf, or 1 tbsp dried

1 handful fresh chickweed (*Stellaria media*) aerial parts

1 cup shiitake (*Lentinula edodes*) mushroom, thinly sliced

1 tbsp ground turmeric (*Curcuma longa*) rhizome

1 tsp sea salt

1 tsp black pepper (*Piper nigrum*) fruit, ground

2 tbsp lemon or lime juice, optional

1. Warm olive oil in a large stock pot and sauté onion for about 5 minutes.
2. Add the chopped ginger rhizome and garlic. Add sliced carrots and parsnips. Cook for a few more minutes, stirring constantly to prevent the garlic from burning.
3. Include the red clover, burdock root and broth. Reduce to a simmer after covering and bringing to a boil. Simmer for half an hour.
4. Use a blender to blend, if desired.
5. Add kale, cabbage, nettle, chickweed and mushrooms, and simmer for another 15 minutes. Add more broth as needed.
6. Add turmeric, sea salt and black pepper. Stir to combine then simmer for 5 minutes more.
7. Serve in a bowl with cooked barley or quinoa, if desired.
8. Add a squeeze of lemon or lime.

Liver support salad

1 pound spring greens

1 handful dandelion (*Taraxacum officinale*) leaf

1 handful chickweed (*Stellaria media*) aerial parts

1 handful violet (*Viola* spp.) leaf

10 violet (*Viola* spp.) flowers

¼ cup sunflower seeds

2 tsp ground milk thistle (*Silybum marianum*) seed or milk thistle gomasio (to taste)

1. Toss all ingredients together in a large bowl.

Safety considerations

No side effects or drug interactions have been reported (Hoffmann, 2003).

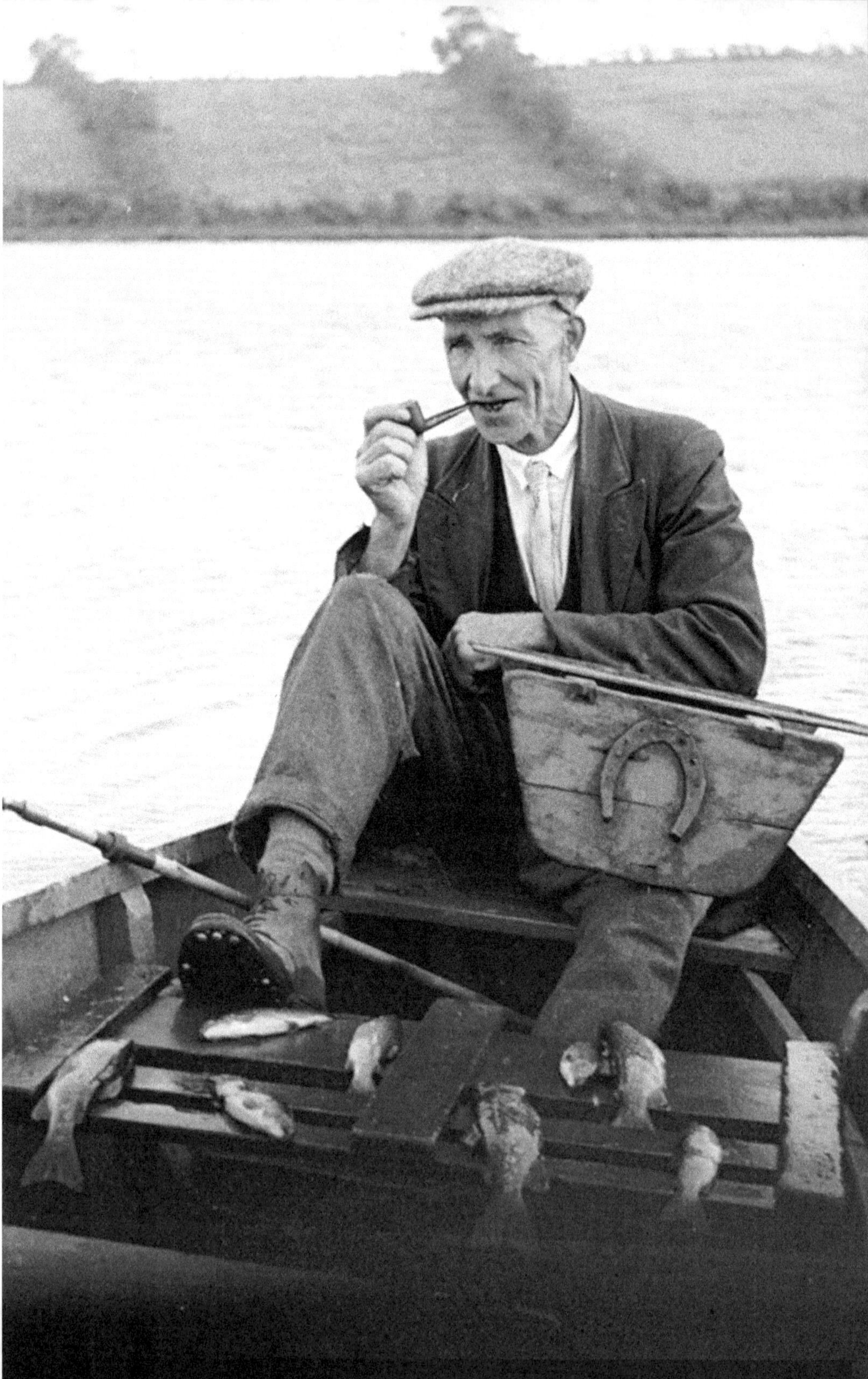

COLTSFOOT

Tussilago farfara

The Schools' Collection, Volume 0057, Page 0123

People all know that they should rub the affected part with dock leaf and strange both it is remarked grow side by side. Dock is a very useful herb and it is so called from the colour of its roots which is the most valuable part of the plant. It is used for hemorrhage of the lungs. The best way of using it as a remedy is, wash roots and boil half a pound of the powdered root in a pint of golden syrup. This can then be taken in teaspoonful doses. It is also used in liver complaints and is a mild laxative. Marshmallow is a nice herb with purple flowers and dark green leaves. The crushed roots will draw out inflammation from boils or wounds when other things fail and it is called Mortification Herb by most country people and when the leaves are brewed (like tea) it is known to cure the most obstinate cough. Coltsfoot, a little of the dried leaves put on a plate and lighted will gradually smoulder away and the smoke inhaled.

The Schools' Collection, Volume 0057, Page 0124

[Coltsfoot] will have a wonderfully healing effect on a sore or inflamed throat or even inflamed lungs. It is always gathered where there is a large family and the leaves are brewed and allowed to stand in a jar or bottle and the liquid is drunk. It is a preventative of colds and chills and is excellent for the most stubborn of coughs.
Chamomile Flowers
Boil flowers and use water for swellings of the face in cases of abscesses, bad teeth, etc.
Milk Weed
Milk weed is a sure cure for warts, break stem, and rub juice or milk to wart after rubbing a few times wart will be seen to decay.
Rose Noble
A weed cure for the mourn in cattle
Cure for Measles
Put child in and out 3 times under the asses belly.
Cure for consumption
Drink the asses milk after foaling

Coughs, colds and chills

The Schools' Collection, Volume 0057, Pages 0123-0124

Coltsfoot, a little of the dried leaves put on a plate and lighted will gradually smoulder away and the smoke inhaled will have a wonderfully healing effect on a sore or inflamed throat or even inflamed lungs. It is always gathered where there is a large family and the leaves are brewed and allowed to stand in a jar or bottle and the liquid is drunk. It is a preventative of colds and chills and is excellent for the most stubborn coughs.

Coltsfoot is best known as a cough soother with an agreeable flavour. Syrups made of the leaf and/or flower are delightful, mild, smooth and slightly minty or honey scented. The Latin genus name Tussilago translates as "cough dispeller", with tussis meaning "cough" and ago meaning "to cast off". It grows in moist places, and flowers at the end of February. It is good for all diseases of the lungs, for coughs, colds, bronchial congestion and consumption. For skin inflammations the leaves pounded with honey can be used (Scott, 1986).

All parts of the plant contain mucilage, long-chain polysaccharides that have a soothing demulcent property (Pengelly, 2004). Mucilage from coltsfoot was found to be as anti-inflammatory as the nonsteroidal anti-inflammatory drug indomethacin (Paine, 2006) and a respiratory stimulant (Paine, 2006). The entire plant also contains inulin, a common constituent of aster family plants that is gently immune-stimulating. Additionally, coltsfoot preparations have been found to have antibacterial effects against certain pathogenic bacteria (Paine, 2006).

Coltsfoot is considered to strengthen and support the respiratory system. The fresh leaves, juice and syrup have been used for dry coughs, wheezing and shortness of breath (Potterton, 2002). The mucilaginous property protects the throat from irritation, reducing cough frequency (van Wyk & Wink, 2014). Coltsfoot dilates the bronchial passages (Tierra, 1998). The overall effect of coltsfoot is moistening and expectorant. Although it is considered a versatile cough herb, it is specifically indicated for convulsive coughing, or stubborn, irritating coughs (Ody, 2017).

In Western herbalism, the leaves are considered particularly anti-inflammatory. The leaves are the part of the plant that are richest in zinc (Hoffmann, 1993), which has been shown to support immune function and reduce inflammation in the mucosal tissue (Haas, 2006; NIH, 2019). Coltsfoot has both an antispasmodic and a calming expectorant effect. Useful amounts of zinc, a mineral with strong anti-inflammatory properties, are present in the leaves. Coltsfoot may aid with asthma, whooping cough, annoying coughs, and acute or chronic bronchitis.

Its soothing expectorant action gives it a role in most respiratory conditions, including emphysema. Priest & Priest described coltsfoot as a diffusive expectorant, sedative and demulcent: suitable for debilitated and chronic conditions (Hoffmann, 2003).

Headache or bad stomach

The Schools' Collection, Volume 0050, Page 0460

The colts-foot grows like shamrock, the only difference being, it's leaves are larger. The leaves are boiled in water for about three quarters of an hour. It is then left to cool and strained and it's juice is like medicine. It is taken for a headache or bad stomach.

This may align with the use in the past of colts-foot for irritation of the gastric mucous membranes and gastric and intestinal catarrh (Felter, 1922).

Coltsfoot – other uses

The leaves also have vulnerary and emollient properties and have been applied topically to boils, abscesses and ulcers (Hoffmann, 1993). For external use, the leaves can be used as a poultice (Rose, 1972) or made into a skin wash by adding 2 cups of mature green leaves to 2 cups of boiling water, then removing from heat to infuse for 1 hour before straining out the herbs and applying the infusion (Brown, 1985). As a mild diuretic, it has been used to treat cystitis (Hoffmann, 2003).

Coltsfoot recipes

Coltsfoot wine

1 litre (5 pints) coltsfoot flowers (*Tussilago farfara*)

1 kg (2¼ lb) sugar

4.5 litres (1 gallon) water

Juice of 2 lemons

Yeast

1. Place the coltsfoot flowers in a plastic bucket.

2. Pour 2 litres (3½ pints) of boiling water on the flowers and leave them to soak for 24 hours, pressing them occasionally with a wooden spoon.

3. Strain off the flowers through muslin, squeezing hard at the end to extract all the flavour.

4. Add the juice of the lemons and the yeast to the bucket

5. Boil the sugar in 2 litres (3½ pints) of water to dissolve it and add it to the bucket.

6. When the liquid has cooled, add the yeast, cover and leave to ferment for 3 days, then transfer to a fermentation jar.

7. Make up the quantity with the rest of the cold boiled water and seal with an airlock.

8. Leave in a warm place 16–20°C (60–70°F) until fermentation has ceased.

9. Then siphon the wine into a clear jar, leaving the main sediment behind.

10. Seal with a cork and leave for a month.

11. Filter the wine to get a sparkling result but if you prefer not to filter it, leave in the jar until the sediment has all settled out and then siphon it off.

12. Bottle and cork with sterilised corks.

Safety considerations

There has been some concern that Tussilago has been found to contain PAs, a harmful group of chemicals that can close off the veins to the liver. The studies have been inadequate and non-conclusive.

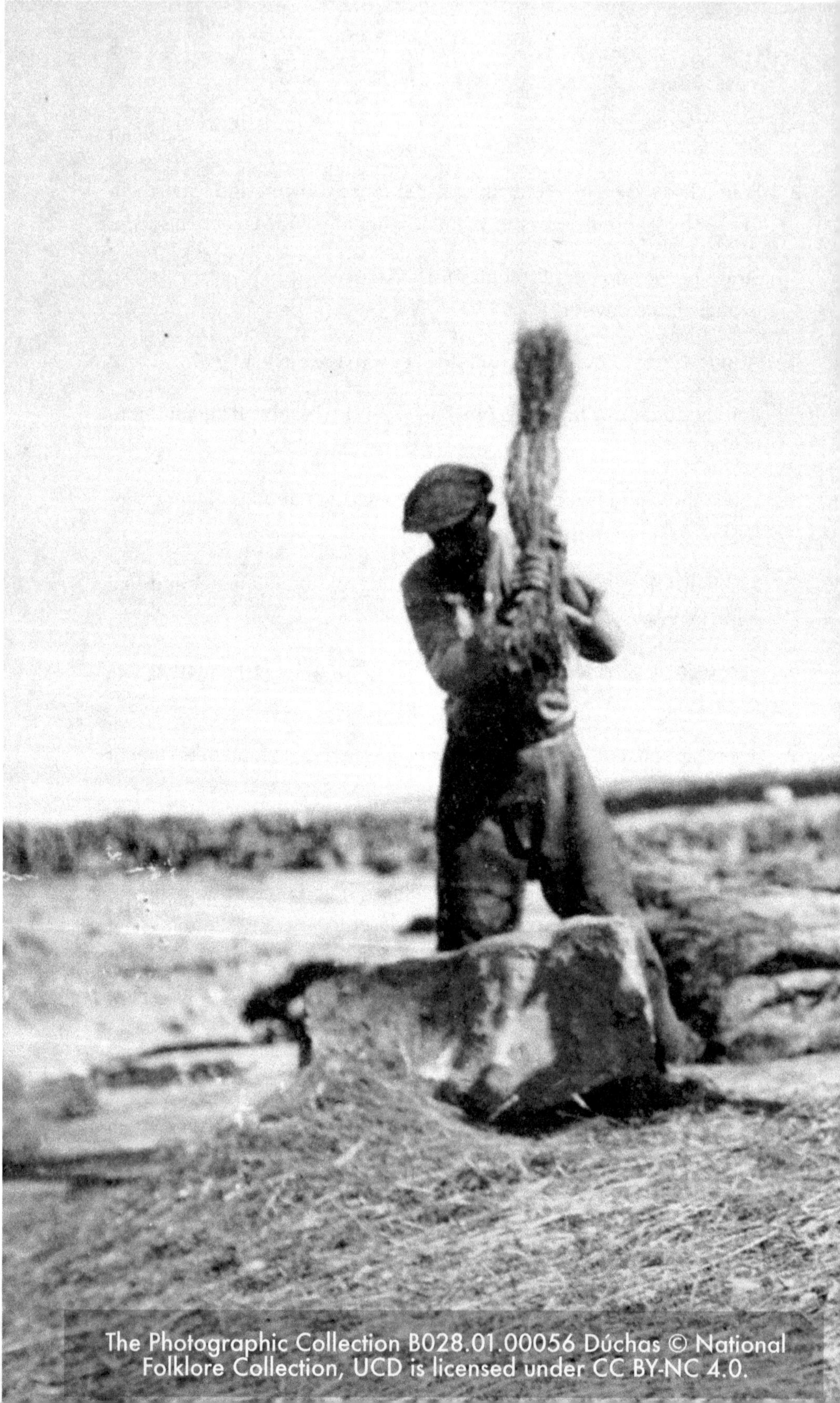

COMFREY

Symphytum officinale

The Schools' Collection, Volume 0050, Page 0401

Cumphery is a cure for sprains.

Alli Compagne is a cure for blood-mourn on cattle and stomach trouble.

Water-cress is a cure for liver trouble.

Drowning leaf is a cure for burns.

Green-Broom is a cure for kidney trouble and a pain in the back.

Dandelion cures lung disease and kidney trouble and is also good for young turkeys

Dock-leaf takes away the pain of a nettle sting.

Hemlock is a cure for Rheumatism, headache and indigestion.

Ivy cures scum in a horses eye and is also used to remove stains.

Bog onion is used to cure pain in the back.

Gladan is a cure for mumps.

Tansey is used to purify the blood and for killing moths.

Fox grass is used for killing worms in cattle.
Nettles are used for curing warts and is also good for ducklings.
Eye-bright is useful in affections of the eyes.
Mostly all of the above are ready for use when boiling water is poured on them.

The Schools' Collection, Volume 0050, Page 0469

The most harmful weed growing on the farm at home is the yellow dock because they spread rapidly and impoverish the land. The thistle is the plant most common that grows on good land. The following are the herbs found on our farm and their cures. Chamomile for nervousness and debility. Dandelion a laxative and a tonic. Clover is used for colds, etc. Comfrey fine medicine for chest complaints also poultices. Red Dock. An excellent blood purifier.

Sprains and poultices

The Schools' Collection, Volume 0050, Page 0401

Cumphery is a cure for sprains.

This use of comfrey is aligned with what we would use comfrey for today. External comfrey preparations such as fomentations and poultices have been used for sprains, swellings and bruises, as well as boils, abscesses and gangrenous ulcers (Grieve, 1931 / 1971). Comfrey leaf is used topically to help with wound healing and to promote proper scar formation. Used as a compress or poultice, comfrey can treat any external ulcers, wounds and fractures and is an excellent treatment for chronic varicose ulcers (Hoffmann, 2003).

In comfrey's botanical name, *Symphytum officinale* the *Symphytum* element translates as "come together", which highlights how well it works to heal wounds.

The constituent responsible for comfrey's vulnerary action is known as allantoin, which stimulates tissue repair and cell proliferation.

Chest complaints

The Schools' Collection, Volume 0050, Page 0469

Comfrey fine medicine for chest complaints also poultices.

Historically, comfrey root or herb has been used for bronchitis and irritable cough to soothe and reduce irritation while promoting expectoration. The mucilage in comfrey is similar to that in marshmallow (*Althaea officinalis*) root, and thus its demulcent action has been used to address everything from whooping cough and consumption to dysentery and diarrhoea (Hoffmann, 2003).

Additionally, historically, comfrey has been used in the healing of ulcerative colitis, hiatus hernias, and gastric and duodenal ulcers. Comfrey's astringency has been used to help haemorrhages and chronic varicose ulcers. Comfrey has been used to help the pancreas in regulating blood sugar levels and to relieve irritations associated with the gallbladder, kidneys, bladder, small intestines and stomach. Comfrey has been used with marshmallow and meadowsweet to treat inflammations and stomach ulcers (Gladstar, 2012). However, as noted below, it is no longer recommended to take Comfrey internally (see "Safety considerations").

Comfrey recipes

Soothing comfrey bath

3 tbsp fresh chopped comfrey or 1½ tbsp dried comfrey (*Symphytum officinale*) leaf

2 cups water

1. Bring water to a boil.

2. Chop the comfrey leaf and place in a pint jar.
3. Pour boiling water over the comfrey and cover.
4. Let the comfrey steep, covered, for 20 minutes to 4 hours.
5. Reserve the liquid for the bath while straining out the herbs.
6. Add the herbal infusion to a warm bath.
7. Relax in the bath for at least 10–20 minutes.

Comfrey oil

300 ml (10 fl oz) olive oil or carrier oil of your choosing

5g (0.2 oz) dried comfrey

How to make a herb-infused oil – two ways

A room temperature herb-infused oil

1. Grind the dried herbs in a mortar and pestle or break them up with your hands to produce smaller pieces.
2. Sterilise a glass jar and fill it halfway with the dried herbs.
3. Cover the dried herbs in the jar almost entirely with room-temperature oil, leaving at least 1 inch of oil above the top of the herbs. To ensure that all of the herb surfaces are covered and there are no air bubbles left, stir well using a clean, dry spoon.
4. To shield the oil from any chemical coating on the lid, place a square piece of natural waxed paper on top of the jar and cover it with a lid.
5. To keep the herb and oil well combined, roll the jar back and forth in your hands.

6. Store the jar in a warm, dark place away from the sun. Give it 4–6 weeks to sit. To assist in mixing the contents and releasing the compounds of the herb into the oil, roll the jar in your palms every one to three days.

7. After 4–6 weeks, decant the oil. In a big bowl with a spout, place a sieve lined with cheesecloth. Fill the strainer with the contents of the jar. Squeeze the remaining oil from the herb into the basin while holding the ends of the cheesecloth together with clean, dry fingertips.

8. Transfer the oil into a glass jar that has been sterilised, cover it, and leave it for a few days or overnight.

9. Strain the oil again, being careful to avoid pouring out any of the remaining herb particulates that have settled to the bottom of the jar.

10. Pour the oil into clean and dry sterilised glass bottles or jars (ideally dark-coloured glass jars to protect from light) and add a few drops of vitamin E oil, if desired, to slow down oxidation of the oil. Cap tightly.

11. Label jar(s) and store in a cool, dark place.

A heated herb-infused oil

1. Add dried herbs to a dry, sanitised heat-safe glass jar. Pour oil over the dried herbs.

2. Leave the lid off the jar without splashing any water into the jar.

3. Place a cloth at the bottom of a slow cooker or saucepan and set the glass jar on top of the cloth. Fill the vessel with enough water to cover to the level of the mixture inside the jar.

4. Set the slow cooker to warm or the stovetop to low heat, the goal being to maintain the water temperature at 120–140° F (49–60° C). Let this

macerate for 4 hours, checking the temperature of the oil regularly to ensure it does not get too hot.

5. Replenish with hot water as necessary to maintain the water level in the slow cooker or saucepan.

6. When time is up, carefully remove the jar from the slow cooker or saucepan and set it aside to cool completely.

7. Place a cheesecloth-lined strainer inside a large dry, sanitised bowl or measuring jug. Pour the contents from the jar into the strainer. With clean, dry hands, gather the ends of the cheesecloth together and squeeze the remaining oil from the herb into the bowl.

8. Pour the oil into a dry, sanitised glass jar, cap, and let it settle overnight.

9. Strain the oil again, being careful to avoid pouring out any of the remaining herb particulates that have settled to the bottom of the jar.

10. Pour the garlic-infused oil into a dry, sanitised glass bottle or jar. Cap tightly and label.

Sprains and strains salve

Use this salve to soothe sprains and strains when the skin is not broken.

4 parts comfrey *(Symphytum officinale)* leaf-infused oil

2 parts yarrow (*Achillea millefolium*) aerial parts-infused oil

2 parts arnica (*Arnica* spp.) flower-infused oil

1 part beeswax (pastilles or grated)

1. See "How to make a herbal infused oil" (pg. 46).

2. Measure the oils and place in a heat-safe bowl over a small saucepan of simmering water over a low heat. Be careful not to splash any water into the oil.

3. Weigh beeswax and add to the warmed oil. Continue to heat the mixture (over a low heat), stirring with a sanitised, dry spoon until the beeswax has melted.

4. While warm, pour individual portions into sanitised salve jars and allow to cool, uncapped, at room temperature.

5. Once cool, put the lids on and label the containers.

6. In a cool, dark place store for up to 1 year.

Safety considerations

Although comfrey has a long history of being used for a variety of purposes, its internal use has become very contentious because of the possibly negative consequences of the herb's pyrrolizidine alkaloids (PAs). It has been demonstrated that PAs in comfrey are carcinogenic in lab animals and hepatotoxic in people and livestock (Mei et al., 2005). The U.S. Food & Drug Administration (FDA) asked for voluntary removal of products containing comfrey in July 2001. Comfrey in oral preparations is banned in Australia, Germany, the United Kingdom and Canada.

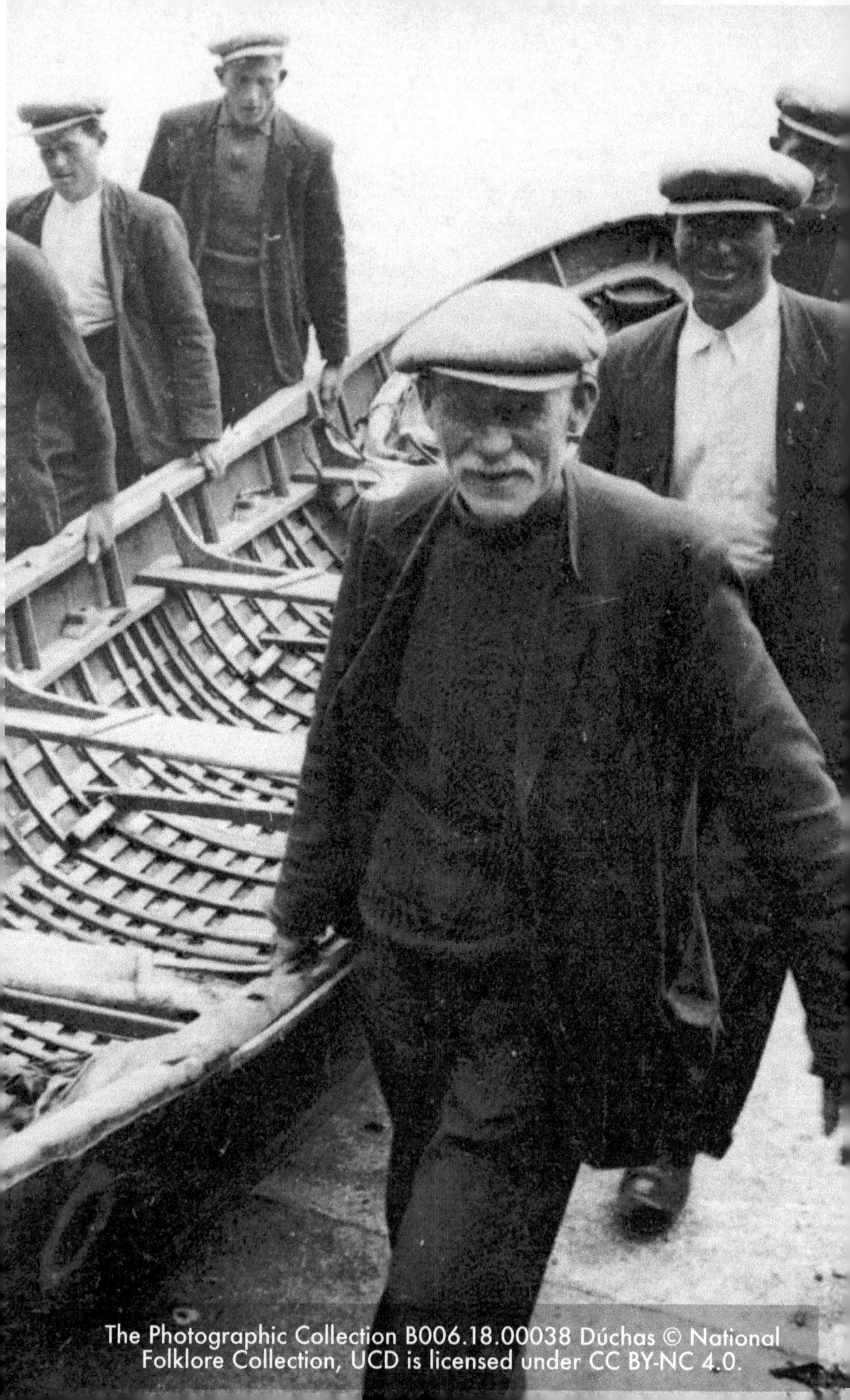

DANDELION

Taraxacum officinale

The Schools' Collection, Volume 0003, Pages 0192 0194

In ancient times when doctors were so few the people had recourse to medicines made from certain herbs to cure their ills. The weeds most harmful on the farm, are the thistle, the fern, the "bráiste" the chicken weed, the nettle and the dock-leaf those impoverish the land. The thistle is the most harmful weed because it grows only on good land and it spreads through the land more than any other weed. The fern also is supposed to grow only on land that produces good potatoe crops. Certain herbs have medicinal properties.

The elderflower and peppermint, taken in hot infusions frequently, is a great remedy for colds and influenza. This infusion is also used as a gargle for sore throats. The watercress when eaten is a wonderful cure for all blood impurities. The cultivated celery which is often used as a vegetable is also most helpful for rheumatic sufferers; it should be stewed well in a little water and taken in doses of two of three tablespoonfuls three times a day.

The common dandelion has also great healing virtues, the plant is of medicinal value and has wonderful purifying properties. It is infused and taken like ordinary coffee with milk and sugar and is a very good cure for kidney and liver disease. Local herbs are used extensively in the cure or alleviation of diseases. In ancient times they were used by the people throughout the country for curing the ills of both people and animals. The dock-leaf is commonly used to cure the sting of a nettle. There is also another leaf called the mason-leaf it is a very good cure both to draw and heal any kind of sore or cut. Nettles are boiled and given to turkeys and other fowl as food, and they are also given to sick calves as a good cure for mourn.

The great majority of people nowadays fail to realise the importance of a knowledge of the laws of good health, and of an knowledge of simple remedies to restore the sick body to health again. These remedies can be obtained from our herbs if properly used.

The Schools' Collection, Volume 0004, Page 0331

Long ago the people made most of the cures from herbs. The dandelion was favourite cure for heart trouble. It was used also for colds. The green leaves of the primrose were put to sores for drawing out.

The Schools' Collection, Volume 0004, Page 0332

Nowadays we hear very little about herbs or their use. There are few people who know about them now. Long ago the people had certain weeds that they used in many ways.

For example they used the green moss that grows on rocks as dye for stockings and other woollen articles. First of all the moss was pulled off the rocks and then it was boiled with the article that was to be coloured. It is still used as a dye in the Islands.

Then there is the chicken-weed which is used to put down swellings or sprains. Water-cress which grows near water is sometimes used as a vegetable. it is also a cure for biles or swelling sores. Old people also say that the duce of the dandelion used to be used as a medicine and now many people use it to get a good complexion. People use the white of a rush to stop blood.

The Schools' Collection, Volume 0004, Page 0333

Some years ago the people were able to distinguish the different herbs, and how to use them as cures for nearly all diseases. Dandelion Slanlis, Crawdan, Garlic water-cress nettles and several others all grow wild nowadays as very few people know and they are never used.
Dandelion was used for the heart, Crawdan and nettles were used for disease. Parsly, thyme and chives are flavouring herbs. The moss that grows on the rocks Scrat-cloc is used for dying woollen good also mader mixed with bog-mud.

The Schools' Collection, Volume 0015, Page 0201

[Nettle-scorches:- a cure for this is] the juice of a dock leaf.
Rheumatism: Dandelion herbs boiled and taken or rubbed of the pain. The dandelion herbs contain milk and they are supposed to cure warts also.
Blood Purifier:- Alder berries bruised and made into wine. The best wine is made from heather. Slow gin is also good for the blood.
Sore ears: Boiled potatoes pressed to the ears.

The Schools' Collection, Volume 0021, Page 0248

Herbs are weeds that grow in fields and gardens. Some of these herbs can cure diseases but others of them are poisonous. God made them I am sure for some purpose.
Here are some of the herbs which can cure diseases. The Garlic or "on Garlóg" was an herb which grew in every garden long ago. It was said that it could cure "Mumps" or swelling around the neck.
The flaggers were herbs that grew in old gardens. It could cure a sore throat. It is a flat herb. These were sown together and put round the place where the throat was sore. This herb was able to cure that disease.

The Awin is also another herb supposed to be able to cure an old burn. This herb grew mostly in old gardens also.
The dandeline is another herb that grows in gardens, fields and other places. It is said that this herb can cure delicacy.
The Rhubarb is also an herb which grows in most gardens. The stalk of this herb is healthy but the leaf of it is poisonous.
The dock-leaf which generally grow in [gardens is also a cure for delicacy. If these are boiled and given to a delicate person it can cure them.]

The Schools' Collection, Volume 0022, Page

Lungs: Dandelion tea - pull the herbs save with sun like hay - draw in teapot like tea - drink the black juice - dress with fruit juices oranges lemons - sugar & raisins & ginger. Good for Liver Limes: A smith in Corofin had a cure for liver trouble. The patient lay on ground smith held sledge in hand & make an apparent attempt to bring it down on patient forcibly. It is said the fright the patient gets watching smith bringing down sledge with terrific force as if were cured the trouble "in se". Smith swung sledge three times. Sean-focal "Bíonn an draoidheacht ar an iarann"

The Schools' Collection, Volume 0029, Page 0358

In mostly every district in Ireland, herbs are to be found in abundance.
A weed called 'chicken weed' causes much harm to the potato crop. It grows in the drills, and robs the potato of the food it needs.
The dandelion is reckoned to be a good cure for Rheumatism. It is boiled, and the juice is rubbed to the places where the Rheumatism has set in.
Another herb is locally called 'The Seven Sisters'. It is called this name, because seven sprouts grow from a long stem. Inside in this stem there is a white milky substance and this is rubbed to warts nine days in succession.
A herb called 'Buglass' is a well known herb in this locality. It has a long stem, large leaves, and a small yellow flower, in the

Season of Spring. The leaves are got and warmed near a fire, then broken into small pieces, and put on a sore foot.

The Schools' Collection, Volume 0040, Page 0105

Dandelion is a cure for liver trouble. Put the dandelions into a pot of water and leave them there until they boil. When the water is boiled take up the pot and strain away the water from the dandelion. Then put the water into a vessel until it cools and then give it to the sick person.

The Schools' Collection, Volume 0045, Page 0067

Dandeline is supposed to be a great medicine in spring. It is good for the liver when boiled, they drink the juice after getting up in the morning.

The Schools' Collection, Volume 0047, Page 0068

Garlic is a small green plant with the bulbous root. The plant is pulled and the tops are cut off.
Two or three garlic roots are then chopped up and put it into a bottle. The bottle is then filled with whiskey and is buried in the clay for nine days. The people use it for a cold or for the whooping cough.
Yarrow is a plant which grows on the road-side near Newtown or in Mr. Barry's land The flower is of a reddish colour with grey spots. This is cut off the stem and chopped up and boiled until it becomes quite soft. Then it is mixed with the juice of a carrot and the old people used it as a cure for sciatica.
The dandelion is great for the lungs. The people pound it and while pounding it they knock the juice out of it. Then they drink it with whiskey.

The Schools' Collection, Volume 0049, Page 0172

Iodine is made from seaweed.
The dandelion has a medicinal property and it is used as a medicine. Dandelion is a medicine and it is supposed to support the heart. Gladum is used for the curing of a sore throat.

The Schools' Collection, Volume 0050, Page 0401

Cumphery is a cure for sprains.
Alli Compagne is a cure for blood-mourn on cattle and stomach trouble.
Water-cress is a cure for liver trouble
Green-Broom is a cure for kidney trouble and a pain in the back.
Dandelion cures lung disease and kidney trouble and is also good for young turkeys

The Schools' Collection, Volume 0050, Pages 0458–0461

Tradition tell us that the people of older times were much healthier than the people are nowadays. The only cure they had for any illness they might have were herbs. They sowed those herbs in gardens, the same as we would sow vegetables now, but the bog-onion grew in bogs, or the banks of some rivers, or streams.

There is not an account of all herbs used in those times. The only ones commonly known are, marsh-mallows, garlic, dandelion, cumfry, chicken-weed, colts-foot, peruvian-bark, bishop's cap, Poppy flowers, camomile flowers, elder, foggy dew and the bog-onion.

The bog-onion resembles a fern in appearance, but its root is somewhat the same as an onion bulb. This root is converted into a juicy substance and used as a rub for rheumatism or sciatica; it is often found to be complete cure. First the root is cut into slices and then pounded up into a mash. It is then put into a bottle or some corked vessel and water supplied in proportion to the size of the root. It is then left to set for about two days until it forms a thick white juicy substance.

The bog onion flowers at night in the month of June, but there is some mystery attached to it, because at the approach of daylight the flower disappears. It is known to be there by leaving seeds after it.

Marsh-mallows grow about three feet high. It is like any ordinary plant and has a pink flower. The roots resemble those of a cabbage plant, and these are boiled in water and their juice is found to be very good for a cold or cough.

The garlic is a bulbous plant of the onion tribe. It's root is pounded into a mash and mixed with lard. It is used as an ointment for sore or tender feet. About half a teaspoonful of this ointment is given on milk to children for the chin-cough.

Dandelion grows flat on the ground with small leaves also inclined to face downwards. It grows a yellow flower. The leaves of the dandelion are boiled with cloves and ginger for about an hour, it is then let cool and strained and afterwards bottled and buried in the ground for about a month. It is then taken up and used. An eggcupful is taken every morning fasting for consumption.

The cumfry grows tall, course, thick leaves about a foot in height. Its flower is purple. Its leaves are pounded and applied for poultices and sprains.

The chicken-weed grows, spread along the ground like moss. It is pounded also and found to be a good cure for chilblains.

The colts-foot grows like shamrock, the only difference being, it's leaves are larger. The leaves are boiled in water for about three quarters of an hour. It is then left to cool and strained and it's juice is like medicine. It is taken for a headache or bad stomach.

Peruvian-bark grows leaves resembling that of a chest-nut. It is boiled in water for about two hours. Then it is left to cool and bottled. It is given to children for rickets.

Bishop's cap is a tall frail plant. It grows about two feet high. Its flower is purple. This flower is boiled in water and used for dyeing purposes.

The poppy is a tender plant and grows about a foot high. Its leaves are boiled and applied as a poultice for the throat.

Camomile flowers are boiled and applied for poultices for the ear. They are found to be the best cure going.

Elder is a high tree its flowers are white. The flowers of it are boiled and mixed with vinegar and camomile flowers; it is applied to wounds and bruises.
The foggy dew is a small plant about a quarter of a foot in height. It makes it first appearance in Spring and disappears again when the season is over. This peculiar little plant is always covered with dew. It is much like heather and is eaten without cooking for diseases of the liver.

The Schools' Collection, Volume 0050, Page 0469

The most harmful weed growing on the farm at home is the yellow dock because they spread rapidly and impoverish the land. The thistle is the plant most common that grows on good land. The following are the herbs found on our farm and their cures. Chamomile for nervousness and debility. Dandelion a laxative and a tonic. Clover is used for colds, etc. Comfrey fine medicine for chest complaints also poultices. Red Dock an excellent blood purifier.

The Schools' Collection, Volume 0057, Page 0122

Dandelion
Its bright yellow flowers must be gathered in the spring from which a brew is made and this is a splendid spring tonic. Its leaves at this time should be dried and bottled in the following way. Spread leaves on a brown paper and put in a slow oven; when crisp and dry take them out and rub between the hands till fine; have a dry hot bottle at hand to put herbs in – cork tightly. Keep in a warm place till required. The roots gathered in the autumn can be washed dried and powdered and thoroughly roasted in the oven till black, this makes excellent coffee and is used by country people as a tonic for liver and kidneys particularly for older people.

The Schools' Collection, Volume 0051, Page 0163

The most harmful weeds in this district are groundsel, crows' foot, nightshade, dandelion robin run the hedge and the thistle – the three last named grow in good land.
Many herbs are used for medicinal purposes The green leaves of the dandelion were eaten for liver complaint. Children collected the leaves which were pounded in a pestle-mortar – a little whiskey was added to the bruised leaves and the mixture was put into a bottle and given to the children to drink.

Kidneys and liver

The Schools' Collection, Volume 0045, Page 0067

Dandeline is supposed to be a great medicine in spring. It is good for the liver when boiled, they drink the juice after getting up in the morning.

The Schools' Collection, Volume 0003, Page 193

The common dandelion has also great healing virtues, the plant is of medicinal value and has wonderful purifying properties. It is infused and taken like ordinary coffee with milk and sugar and is a very good cure for kidney and liver disease.

The Schools' Collection, Volume 0051, Page 0163

The green leaves of the dandelion were eaten for liver complaint. Children collected the leaves which were pounded in a pestle-mortar – a little whiskey was added to the bruised leaves and the mixture was put into a bottle and given to the children to drink.

The Schools' Collection, Volume 0040, Page 0105

Dandelion is a cure for liver trouble. Put the dandelions into a pot of water and leave them there until they boil. When the water is boiled take up the pot and strain away the water from

> the dandelion. Then put the water into a vessel until it cools and then give it to the sick person.

The Schools' Collection, Volume 0057, Page 0122

> Its bright yellow flowers must be gathered in the spring from which a brew is made and this is a splendid spring tonic. Its leaves at this time should be dried and bottled in the following way. Spread leaves on a brown paper and put in a slow oven; when crisp and dry take them out and rub between the hands till fine; have a dry hot bottle at hand to put herbs in - cork tightly. Keep in a warm place till required. The roots gathered in the autumn can be washed dried and powdered and thoroughly roasted in the oven till black, this makes excellent coffee and is used by country people as a tonic for liver and kidneys particularly for older people.

The stimulating impact of dandelion leaf on the kidneys promotes appropriate uric acid clearance, which eliminates metabolic wastes and makes it an excellent diuretic. This helps with rheumatism, arthritis, gout, water retention, and prostate and urinary tract infections. The high potassium and other mineral content of dandelion compensates for the potassium and mineral loss that occurs through urine.

Thus, dandelion is a safe diuretic to use even in the case of water retention associated with cardiac conditions (Hoffmann, 2003).

As a hepatic (supports liver function, aids detoxification, and promotes tissue repair) and cholagogue (stimulates the gallbladder to contract, promoting the flow of bile into the intestines. This action aids in fat digestion, relieves bloating, and helps the body naturally eliminate waste), dandelion root may be helpful for inflammation and congestion of the liver and gallbladder.

Dandelion is a supreme liver tonic as it excels at clearing excess heat (inflammation), clearing stagnation (congestion), and supporting detoxification of metabolic wastes.

Dandelion stimulates the gallbladder, has an affinity with the liver, and helps reduce congestion and inflammation in both organs (Hoffmann, 2003). According to McIntyre (1996), it is used to treat gallbladder infections, jaundice, liver illness, acute hepatitis and dissolving gallstones. Additionally, it is regarded as an alterative, helping the liver eliminate metabolic wastes from the blood, so clearing up eruptive skin problems such as eczema. Dandelion "encourages the eliminative changes carried on by the liver", according to Ellingwood (1919).

Skin and warts

The Schools' Collection, Volume 0004, Page 0332

Old people also say that the duce of the dandelion used to be used as a medicine and now many people use it to get a good complexion. People use the white of a rush to stop blood.

The Schools' Collection, Volume 0015, Page 0201

Rheumatism:- Dandelion herbs boiled and taken or rubbed of the pain. The dandelion herbs contain milk and they are supposed to cure warts also.

The Schools' Collection, Volume 0046, Page 0113

Dandelion herbs contain milk and they are supposed to cure warts also.

Dandelion has certainly been recognised as a topical remedy for warts and for skin issues. Ellingwood recommended dandelion root for chronic skin eruptions (Hoffmann, 2003).

The white, milky sap in the stem of dandelion is a natural latex that effectively dissolves warts when applied topically (Bennett, 2014). Those with a latex allergy should proceed cautiously and do a skin patch test first (Hoffmann, 2003).

Tonic

The Schools' Collection, Volume 0021, Page 0248

The dandeline is another herb that grows in gardens, fields and other places. It is said that this herb can cure delicacy.

The Schools' Collection, Volume 0050, Page 0459

Dandelion grows flat on the ground with small leaves also inclined to face downwards. It grows a yellow flower. The leaves of the dandelion are boiled with cloves and ginger for about an hour, it is then let cool and strained and afterwards bottled and buried in the ground for about a month. It is then taken up and used. An eggcupful is taken every morning fasting for consumption.

The Schools' Collection, Volume 0050, Page 0469

Dandelion a laxative and a tonic.

Dandelion is an excellent mild bitter tonic and balances the sweet and salty taste addictions of a stressed-out Western culture in chronic flight-or-fight mode. Bitter herbs such as dandelion help to stimulate appetite and activate digestion and metabolism by stimulating secretion of bile, gastric enzymes and pancreatic enzymes. Dandelion root increases the amount of bile produced by the liver and gallbladder, aiding the digestion of fats (Tillotson, 2001).

David Hoffmann (2003) calls dandelion "a most valuable general tonic and perhaps the best widely applicable diuretic and liver tonic". It is this value as a general tonic that may explain the wide-ranging references to the use of dandelion.

The Schools' Collection, Volume 0022, Page 0238

Lungs: Dandelion tea - pull the herbs save with sun like hay - draw in teapot like tea - drink the black juice - dress with fruit juice oranges - lemons - sugar & raisins & ginger.

The Schools' Collection, Volume 0047, Page 0068

The dandelion is great for the lungs. The people pound it and while pounding it they knock the juice out of it. Then they drink it with whiskey.

The Schools' Collection, Volume 0050, Page 0401

Dandelion cures lung disease and kidney trouble and is also good for young turkeys

The Schools' Collection, Volume 0004, Page 0331

The dandelion was favourite cure for heart trouble. It was used also for colds.

The Schools' Collection, Volume 0004, Page 0333

Dandelion was used for the heart.

The Schools' Collection, Volume 0049, Page 0172

The dandelion has a medicinal property and it is used as a medicine. Dandelion is a medicine and it is supposed to support the heart.

Rheumatism

The Schools' Collection, Volume 0029, Page 0358

The dandelion is reckoned to be a good cure for Rheumatism. It is boiled, and the juice is rubbed to the places where the Rheumatism has set in.

In addition, this reference reflects the fact that dandelion can be very effective as part of a wider treatment for muscular rheumatism. Dandelion root has been recommended by Ellingwood for rheumatism (Hoffmann, 2023).

Dandelion leaves have long been used as a mild diuretic for water retention and bladder/kidney problems. Unlike synthetic diuretics, dandelion is high in potassium and replenishes rather than depletes this important nutrient in the system.

Dandelion is one of the best herbs for detoxification. The roots are a classic "liver tonic" or "blood purifier", aiding in optimising digestion by filtering and removing wastes from the bloodstream. The roots (and leaves) are rich in bitter compounds that stimulate receptor sites on the tongue, which then send signals to the digestive tract. The roots also have a beneficial effect on the gallbladder by stimulating bile production, which in turn helps break down cholesterol and fat.

The root has a stimulating and decongestant effect on the liver, making it a traditional liver tonic or blood purifier. In addition to stimulating the kidneys to eliminate toxins from the urine, it primarily acts on the liver and gallbladder to aid in the removal of waste products. Dandelion is beneficial for a wide range of ailments, such as gout, osteoarthritis, psoriasis, eczema and acne, as well as constipation.

Both dandelion root and leaf have been used to prevent gallstones. The leaf may also help dissolve already formed gallstones. Dandelion helps decrease high blood pressure, which in turn aids the action of the heart and is believed to help with anaemia (Gladstar, 2012).

Dandelion is an alterative. Alteratives improve the metabolic functioning of the body. Alteratives have been defined as acting through the lymphatic, glandular and mucous membrane systems to favourably alter the breakdown and elimination of metabolic waste (Smith, 2008)

Alterative plants also nourish the body and support the assimilation of nutrients. Alteratives act by feeding and nourishing the body – by supporting it – rather than by forcing it to behave in one manner or another. Therefore, these herbs are more akin to nourishing foods than medicines (Hoffmann, 2003). Dandelion leaves can be made into salads or a dandelion root tincture can be taken 20 minutes before a meal to support digestion as well and ease indigestion and constipation. Owing to its gentle improvement of bile flow, dandelion acts as a mild laxative (Tillotson, 2001). Dandelion is bitter, so it can be blended with milder herbs.. The leaves can also be infused for tea (Gladstar, 2012). The root, when tender, can also be chopped and added to stir-fries and soups.

The bitter greens of dandelion are rich in iron, calcium, potassium, vitamins and a rich assortment of trace minerals. Dandelions can be steamed, often with other wild greens, and served drizzled with olive oil and lemon juice. The flowers can be made into a delicious wine or gently sautéed in butter for a fine crunchy flavour reminiscent of fried mushrooms. The flowers and stalks contain milky latex, which is helpful in getting rid of warts: apply the fresh milky latex directly on the wart several times daily for two to three weeks. If there is a reaction to the latex or a rash develops, discontinue use.

The root is often roasted and used as a rich flavourful tea, frequently referred to as a "coffee substitute". Heavy roasting, however, will destroy some of the medicinal properties. Combine the heavily roasted dandelion with the raw root half and half, for the medicinal properties of the raw root mixed with the flavourful properties of the root when roasted.

Dandelion root is frequently decocted and used as a liver tonic tea. Its mildly bitter flavour can be easily enhanced by combining it with other herbs that have more flavour. The root can be sliced and pickled and when tender can also be added to stir-fries and soups.

Dandelion recipes

Marinated dandelion greens

[Adapted from Rosemary Gladstar's book *Herbal Recipes for Vibrant Health.*]

Dandelion greens (*Taraxacum officinale*)

<u>Dressing ingredients:</u>

1 part olive oil

1 part vinegar or lemon juice

Garlic to taste

Honey to taste

Culinary herbs of your choosing, like thyme and basil

Toasted sesame oil optional

1. Make a marinade sauce of equal parts virgin olive oil and vinegar. Add honey, garlic, the herbs of your choice such as thyme and basil and pepper to flavour.

2. Steam the dandelion greens and drain any liquid from them. Allow to cool.

3. Pour the dressing over the greens and let them marinate at least overnight.

Wild herb casserole with dandelion greens

¼ cup butter

Onions

3–4 quarts dandelion (*Taraxacum officinale*) and in-season fresh herb greens such as amaranth, lambs' quarters or nettle

1 cup milk or water

4 eggs

¾ cup flour

Grated cheese

Seasonings such as salt, pepper, curry, Italian spices, etc.

1. Place butter in the bottom of a 6 x 10 inch baking dish.

2. Turn the oven on to 425° F (220° C) and melt the butter in the pan.

3. Sauté onion(s) in the pan until golden brown and tender. Add chopped fresh herbs. Sauté until soft and well cooked. Drain off any liquid.

4. While herbs are cooking, place the following ingredients in the blender and blend until creamy: milk (or water), eggs, flour and seasonings.

5. Place the sautéed herbs in the baking dish. Cover the herbs with grated cheese.

6. Pour the egg–milk mixture over it.

7. Bake for 30 to 45 minutes. It is done when a knife inserted in the middle comes out clean. Serve immediately or cool and serve later.

Dandelion and burdock tincture

Fresh dandelion root (*Taraxacum officinale*)

Fresh burdock root (*Arctium lappa*)

Alcohol (brandy, gin or vodka)

1. Gather fresh dandelion roots and burdock roots, clean and chop finely (dried roots can be used). Place in a wide-mouth canning jar and cover with just enough alcohol (brandy, gin or vodka) so that roots are completely covered by an inch or two of liquid. Cover tightly and leave in a warm place for 4–6 weeks.

2. Shake daily to keep the herbs mixing with the alcohol. Strain and rebottle when finished. Label with name, date and ingredients.

3. To use: take ½–1 tsp three times a day.

Dandelion mocha

3 cups water

3 tbsp roasted dandelion roots (*Taraxacum officinale*)

1 tbsp raw cocoa nibs or raw chocolate

½ cup milk or almond milk

½ tsp powdered cinnamon

½ tsp pure vanilla extract

1 tbsp maple syrup or honey

Dash of nutmeg powder or clove

1. Place the roasted dandelion root and cocoa nibs (or unsweetened chocolate) in a pot and cover them with the cold water.

2. Place the pot on the stove over medium-high heat and bring the mixture to a slow, rolling boil.

3. Immediately reduce the heat to low, cover the pot with a lid, and let it gently simmer.

4. Simmer for 20 to 40 minutes or until the liquid has reduced to about half or two-thirds of its original volume.

5. Remove the pot from the heat. Place a muslin cloth or a fine-mesh sieve over a heatproof jug and pour the liquid through it. Squeeze any excess moisture from the herbs.

6. Add the remaining ingredients, stir and heat again if necessary. Top with a dash of nutmeg powder.

Dandelion vinegar

2 to 3 dandelion plants, including roots, stems, leaves and flowers (*Taraxacum officinale*)

Enough cider vinegar to cover the plants in a pint-size jar

1. Soak your dandelions in a bowl of cold water, rinsing any dirt from the roots and leaves.
2. Finely chop, including the stems and leaves.
3. Place the dandelions in a clean pint-size glass jar, filling the jar at least halfway with them.
4. Pour cider vinegar all the way to the top of the jar and use a knife to stir it all together, making sure everything is well covered in vinegar.
5. Cover the mouth of the jar with a square of parchment paper and screw the lid on over the paper.
6. Label your jar with the name and date.
7. Give it a little shake and leave in a dark space for at least 1 week, and up to 2 months. Strain out the dandelion plant material, reserving the vinegar and pouring it back into your jar.
8. This vinegar can be used in dressings, sauces, sparkling water or soups.

Dandelion root beer

1 tbsp dandelion (*Taraxacum officinale*) root

⅛ tsp cinnamon (*Cinnamomum verum*) bark flakes (avoid using powder)

½ tsp fresh or dried ginger (*Zingiber officinale*)

Small handful of mashed raisins (recommended)

Water

1 small bottle of sparkling water

1. Place herbs and (if using) mashed raisins or crystallised ginger into a tea pot, coffee press or canning jar.
2. Add boiling water.
3. Let infuse until herbal infusion returns to room temperature.
4. Once cool, taste. If not fizzy enough for your taste, add the sparking water.

Liver support coffee substitute

¼ cup dandelion (*Taraxacum officinale*) root

¼ cup burdock (*Arctium lappa*) root

½ cup chicory (*Cichorium intybus*) root

½ tbsp cinnamon (*Cinnamomum* spp.) bark, powdered

1 tbsp cacao powder

1. Preheat the oven to 375° F (190° C).
2. Spread the dandelion, burdock and chicory root on a baking sheet and bake 20 minutes and the roots have turned a darker shade of brown.

3. Remove from the oven and let cool.

4. After the herbs have cooled, add them to a coffee grinder and grind into a fine powder.

5. Spread the powder on the baking sheet and bake at 325° F for another 5 minutes.

6. Remove from the oven and let cool.

7. Add the cinnamon and cacao powder to the tray and stir to combine, then transfer to a clean and labelled glass jar with lid.

8. To use, add 3 heaping tbsp to your French press or coffee maker. Add 12 fl oz boiling water, steep for 5 minutes, strain and add milk of choice or honey (or sweetener of choice) if desired.

Liver support tincture

Restores the liver and promotes healthy and natural liver detoxification. Helpful if you feel drained and tired

½ fl oz dandelion (*Taraxacum officinale*) root, tincture or glycerite

½ fl oz burdock (*Arctium lappa*) root, tincture or glycerite

½ fl oz milk thistle (*Silybum marianum*) seed, tincture or glycerite

½ fl oz reishi (*Ganoderma lucidum*) mushroom, tincture or glycerite

1. Measure ingredients into a small, clean bowl or measuring jar and stir to combine.

2. Transfer to a 2 fl oz dropper bottle for daily use.

3. Have 20 drops up to 2 times per day.

Safety considerations

Dandelion may theoretically cause allergic reactions in people sensitive to plants in the Asteraceae family. There have been rare reports of contact dermatitis in people coming in frequent contact with the latex found in the stem (Hoffmann, 2003).

DOCK LEAF

Rumex crispus

The Schools' Collection, Volume 0021, Pages 0248-0249

Herbs are weeds that grow in fields and gardens. Some of these herbs can cure diseases but others of them are poisonous. God made them I am sure for some purpose.
Here are some of the herbs which can cure diseases. The Garlic or "on Garlóg" was an herb which grew in every garden long ago. It was said that it could cure "Mumps" or swelling around the neck.
The flaggers were herbs that grew in old gardens. It could cure a sore throat. It is a flat herb. These were sown together and put round the place where the throat was sore. This herb was able to cure that disease.
The Awin is also another herb supposed to be able to cure an old burn. This herb grew mostly in old gardens also.
The dandeline is another herb that grows in gardens, fields and other places. It is said that this herb can cure delicacy.

The Rhubarb is also an herb which grows in most gardens. The stalk of this herb is healthy but the leaf of it is poisonous.
The dock-leaf which generally grow [in gardens is also a cure for delicacy. If these are boiled and given to a delicate person it can cure them.]

The Schools' Collection, Volume 0021, Pages 0248–0249

The dock-leaf which generally grow in gardens is also a cure for delicacy. If these are boiled and given to a delicate person it can cure

The Schools' Collection, Volume 0046, Page 0197

A cure for warts is to rub the juice of a dandelion of them. A cure for the whooping cough is to take ferret's leavings seven times after one another. Dock leaves boiled and eaten in spring purifies the blood. The garlic is a cure for ring worm and boils. The camomile is a cure for rheumatism. To rub a snail of a wart and then to hang the snail up on gooseberry will the wart.

The Schools' Collection, Volume 0050, Page 0470

Yellow Dock – for rheumatism and liver trouble.
Nettle Seed – Useful in chest infections and as a blood medicine.
Ash Leaves – Useful in cases of gout and rheumatism.
There is moss growing in Loughatorick and it is used by the women there for dyeing flannel.

The Schools' Collection, Volume 0057, Page 0123

People all know that they should rub the affected part with dock leaf and strange both it is remarked grow side by side. Dock is a very useful herb and it is so called from the colour of its roots which is the most valuable part of the plant. It is used for hemorrhage of the lungs. The best way of using it as a remedy is, wash roots and boil half a pound of the powdered root in a pint of golden syrup. This can then be taken in teaspoonful doses. It is also used in liver complaints and is a mild laxative. Marshmallow is a nice herb with purple flowers and dark green leaves. The crushed roots will draw out inflammation from boils or wounds when other things fail and it is called Mortification Herb by most country people and when the leaves are brewed (like tea) it is known to cure the most obstinate cough. Coltsfoot, a little of the dried leaves put on a plate and lighted will gradually smoulder away and the smoke inhaled

The Schools' Collection, Volume 0077, Page 0064

There are not as many cures now as there were long ago.
My Grandmother told me a few.
(1) Nettles are very good to eat during the month of March, and it is said that you should boil them and eat them three times during the month, and the person that does this will not get any disease during the year.
(2) The roots of docket leaves boiled in milk are used to cure a sick stomach.
(3) Garlic boiled in milk is good for a cold, and to put some into your shoes would cure rheumatism.

Tonic

The Schools' Collection, Volume 0021, Pages 0248–0249

The dock-leaf which generally grow in gardens is also a cure for delicacy. If these are boiled and given to a delicate person it can cure them.

The reference to delicacy suggests a need for a tonic, and yellow dock is an obvious choice in this regard. Yellow dock is high in a variety of vitamins and minerals such as calcium, magnesium, manganese, phosphorus and vitamin A. Historically used for scurvy, the plant also contains ample vitamin C (Pedersen, 1998; Wood, 2008). Owing to its high iron content and capacity to enhance iron absorption, yellow dock has also been used to treat anaemia. Thus, it is helpful to combine yellow dock with other iron-rich foods, such as nettle and seaweed, for the most benefit (Katz, 2016). One traditional remedy is yellow dock syrup, made by combining a root decoction with molasses, honey, or maple syrup (Angier, 2008; Hoffelt, 2016).

The dock root is an easily digested form of bio-chelated iron which your body can readily absorb. Dock root has been used for anaemia and fatigue and may be useful for hormonal issues (Gladstar, 2012).

Blood

The Schools' Collection, Volume 0046, Page 0197

Dock leaves boiled and eaten in spring purifies the blood.

This is likely owing to yellow dock's alterative properties, and in folk medicine yellow dock is often called a "blood purifier" or "blood cleanser". Several Native American tribes, such as the Cherokee, Delaware, Iroquois, Mohegan, Paiute and Shoshoni, also have a history of using yellow dock to purify the blood and ease a variety of ailments (Moerman, 2009). Physiomedical and Eclectic physicians classified the plant as an alterative, employing it in cases of "bad blood" associated with skin conditions and glandular congestion (Cook, 1869; Ellingwood, 1919; Lloyd & Felter, 1898).

Liver and digestion

The Schools' Collection, Volume 0077, Page 0064

There are not as many cures now as there were long ago.
My Grandmother told me a few.
(1) Nettles are very good to eat during the month of March, and it is said that you should boil them and eat them three times during the month, and the person that does this will not get any disease during the year.

(2) The roots of docket leaves boiled in milk are used to cure a sick stomach.
(3) Garlic boiled in milk is good for a cold, and to put some into your shoes would cure rheumatism.

The Schools' Collection, Volume 0057, Page 0123

[When stung with a nettle the country] people all know that they should rub the affected part with dock leaf and strange both it is remarked grow side by side. Dock is a very useful herb and it is so called from the colour of its roots which is the most valuable part of the plant. It is used for hemorrhage of the lungs. The best way of using it as a remedy is, wash roots and boil half a pound of the powdered root in a pint of golden syrup. This can then be taken in teaspoonful doses. It is also used in liver complaints and is a mild laxative.

The Schools' Collection, Volume 0050, Page 0470

Yellow Dock – for rheumatism and liver trouble.

The reference to the use of yellow dock in the context of the liver and digestion is understandable. Yellow dock has a strong affinity for the digestive system and is an important digestive ally. The bitter qualities of the plant stimulate the gallbladder and liver, facilitate fat digestion and nutritional absorption, and shorten the time it takes for the stool to pass. The cooling qualities of yellow dock also reduce gastrointestinal tract inflammation (Katz, 2016).

Laxative

Yellow dock root is rich in anthraquinone, which provides a laxative action. According to Guido Masé (2013), "there is no safer or gentler bitter when it comes to ensuring regular bowel function" (p. 178). He uses a tincture of yellow dock in combination with a diet high in fibre and bitter greens for clients who have become dependent upon over-the-counter laxatives for bowel movements. He also suggests yellow dock for easing constipation that can occur during travel and pregnancy (Masé, 2013). Yellow dock has been used in cases of constipation caused by side effects of prescription drugs (Klenner, 2016).

Yellow dock – other uses

Additionally, yellow dock is often used to treat psoriasis and other chronic skin conditions. Yellow dock was regarded by Priest & Priest as a "general tonic alterative with special action upon skin eruptions" (Hoffmann, 2003).

Dock leaf recipes

Iron rich root tonic

[Adapted from Robin Rose Bennett, *The Gift of Healing Herbs*]

1 cup dried burdock root (*Arctium lappa*)

½ cup dried dandelion root (*Taraxacum officinale*)

½ cup dried yellow dock root (*Rumex crispus*)

½ cup dried nettle leaf (*Urtica dioica*)

6 tbsp molasses

1. Add herbs to a half-gallon jar, fill jar with boiling water, and cap.
2. Let infuse for 8–12 hours, then strain.
3. Pour the infusion into a pot and cook until the volume has been cut in half. Cut off the heat and let it cool.
4. Combine molasses and decoction, pour into a jar, and cover.
5. The tonic will keep for one to two months in the refrigerator. As needed, take 2 tbsp twice a day.

Blood building tonic

3g (0.10 oz) codonopsis (*Codonopsis pilosula*) root

2g (0.07 oz) goji (*Lycium* spp.) berry

2g (0.07 oz) oat (*Avena sativa*) straw or milky seed

2g (0.07 oz) nettle leaf (*Urtica dioica*)

0.5g (0.02 oz) yellow dock (*Rumex crispus*) root

0.5g (0.02 oz) cinnamon (*Cinnamomum* spp.) bark

0.5g (0.02 oz) cardamom (*Elettaria cardamomum*) seed

0.5g (0.02 oz) orange (*Citrus* spp.) peel

1. Place 0.75L–1L (24–32 fl oz) water in a small saucepan with the herbs.
2. Bring to a boil, then lower heat and simmer for 20 minutes, covered.
3. Turn off the heat and strain the decoction into a drinking vessel.
4. Add milk of choice or honey (or sweetener of choice) if desired.
5. Drink throughout the day, and store any remaining decoction in the refrigerator for up to 48 hours.

Safety considerations

Children or people who are pregnant or breastfeeding should not use large quantities of yellow dock (Kuhn & Winston, 2008).

Fresh yellow dock root may cause vomiting, and may potentiate the activity of stimulant laxatives (Hoffmann, 2003).

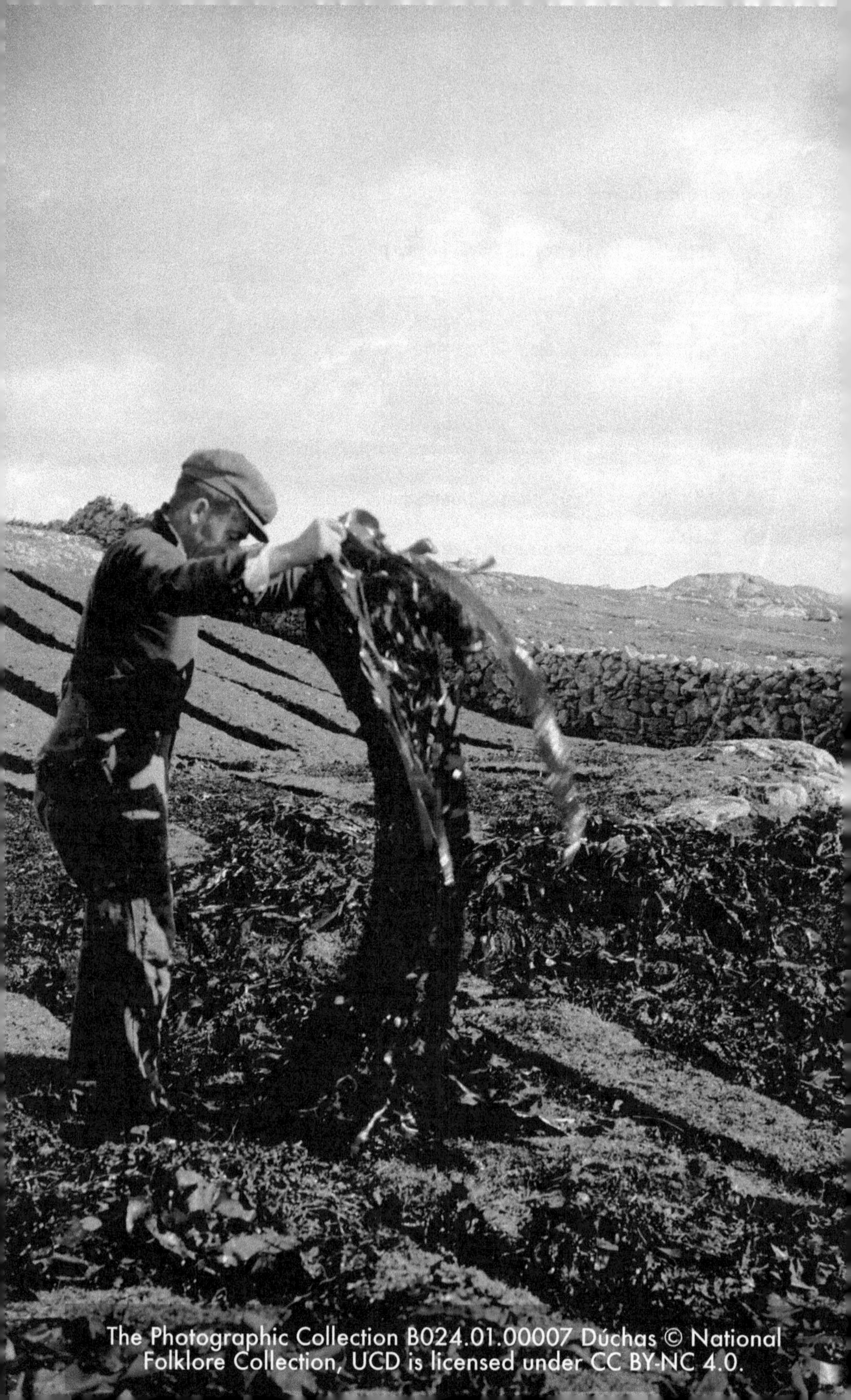

ELDER

Sambucus nigra

The Schools' Collection, Volume 0003, Page 0192

In ancient times when doctors were so few the people had recourse to medicines made from certain herbs to cure their ills. The weeds most harmful on the farm, are the thistle, the fern, the "bráiste" the chicken weed, the nettle and the dock-leaf those impoverish the land. The thistle is the most harmful weed because it grows only on good land and it spreads through the land more than any other weed. The fern also is supposed to grow only on land that produces good potatoe crops. Certain herbs have medicinal properties.

The elderflower and peppermint, taken in hot infusions frequently, is a great remedy for colds and influenza. This infusion is also used as a gargle for sore throats.

The Schools' Collection, Volume 0015, Page 0201

[Nettle-scorches:- a cure for this is] the juice of a dock leaf.

Rheumatism:- Dandelion herbs boiled and taken or rubbed of the pain. The dandelion herbs contain milk and they are supposed to cure warts also. Blood Purifier:- Alder berries bruised and made into wine. The best wine is made from heather. Slow-gin is also good for the blood. Sore ears:- Boiled potatoes pressed to the ears.

The Schools' Collection, Volume 0050, Pages 0460–0461

Elder is a high tree, its flowers are white. The flowers of it are boiled and mixed with vinegar and camomile flowers; it is applied to wounds and bruises.

The foggy dew is a small plant about a quarter of a foot in height. It makes it first appearance in Spring and disappears again when the season is over. This peculiar little plant is always covered with dew. Hence it gets the name of the foggy dew. It is much like heather and is eaten without cooking for diseases of the liver.

The Schools' Collection, Volume 0057, Page 0121

Herbs were introduced it is commonly believed by the monks who established monasteries over the country thousands of years ago and was used with great advantage by the old monks who had a cure for almost every disease, one of their greatest being Common Elder Flowers.

Elder flowers may be gathered in the early Spring or Summer and from them an infusion may be made (like tea) one ounce of dried flowers should be infused in one pint of hot water this will speedily cure croup or suffocation in children or for "Grown Ups" who contract a cold during the day if they take a half tea cupful hot going to bed, will rid themselves of a cold or fever by the next morning. Old men in the country on a summer's day wear it in their hats whilst others rub it over their face and hands to keep away swarms of insects, who would sting or bite them. Dried elder flowers are dull yellow in colour are an excellent drink in summer or winter as it is a mild aperient and it is given in cases of no clearly defined illness.

Colds and flu

The Schools' Collection, Volume 0003, Page 0192

The elderflower and peppermint, taken in hot infusions frequently, is a great remedy for colds and influenza. This infusion is also used as a gargle for sore throats.

The Schools' Collection, Volume 0057, Page 0121

Elder flowers may be gathered in the early Spring or Summer and from them an infusion may be made (like tea) one ounce of dried flowers should be infused in one pint of hot water this will speedily cure croup or suffocation in children or for "Grown Ups" who contract a cold during the day if they take a half tea cupful hot going to bed, will rid themselves of a cold or fever by the next morning. Old men in the country on a summer's day wear it in their hats whilst others rub it over their face and hands to keep away swarms of insects, who would sting or bite them. Dried elder flowers are dull yellow in colour are an excellent drink in summer or winter as it is a mild aperient and it is given in cases of no clearly defined illness.

Owing to their diaphoretic and antiviral properties, elderflower and elderberry – referred to as a "medicine chest in its own right" (Hoffmann, 2003) – are both great allies during colds, the flu and respiratory infections. Both are suitable for use in children; the flavour of black elderberry syrup is pleasant and beneficial in flu cases, and the blooms can be used with peppermint or spearmint in a tea to help lower fevers (Romm, 2024).

Elderflower is particularly regarded for its capacity to expedite recovery and ease flu symptoms (Easley & Horne, 2016).

Additionally, elderflower has anti-inflammatory, anti-catarrhal and expectorant properties. It also helps to reduce sinus tissue inflammation and facilitate congestion movement in cases of colds, sinusitis and sinus allergies. Elderberry also helps with congestion and coughing brought on by viral infections of the lower respiratory tract, encouraging the expectoration of mucus from bronchial infections. Elderberries are also known to help prevent the spread of viruses (Easley & Horne, 2016).

Elder is an immune stimulant, rather than an immunomodulatory; the immune-stimulating impact is thought to be associated with the regulatory influence the berries exert on cytokines (chemicals released into the blood during illness) (Heckels et al., 2019). Traditionally, the berries were used to craft homemade wine or cordials and taken hot with sugar right before bedtime to ward off colds and bronchitis (Grieve, 1971).

Blood purifier

The Schools' Collection, Volume 0015, Page 020

Blood Purifier:- Alder berries bruised and made into wine.

As an alterative, elderflower aids in enhancing the expulsion and elimination of metabolic wastes, proving helpful in instances of oedema (Smith, 2008). The emmenagogue properties of the berries also enhance blood circulation to the pelvic region, potentially inducing delayed menses (Heckels et al., 2019).

Wounds and bruises

The Schools' Collection, Volume 0050, Pages 0460–0461

Elder is a high tree its flowers are white. The flowers of it are boiled and mixed with vinegar and camomile flowers; it is applied to wounds and bruises.

This also aligns with the lesser-known use of elder tree leaf topically for bruises, sprains, wounds and chilblains (Hoffmann, 2003). Fresh elder leaf is used externally as a poultice or an oil infusion for bruises, sprains and wounds through its vulnerary (tissue supportive) and astringent (toning) actions. The leaves also aid skin issues from infections to swelling to burns (Salmón, 2020). Herbalist Richo Cech (2016) suggests creating an infused herbal oil using the fresh, green leaves; this oil can be applied as is or transformed into a refreshing green salve or cream. Cech (2016) shares that oily formulations from fresh elder leaf prove beneficial in cases of traumatic injuries or old burns (Grieve, 1971).

Elder recipes

Elderberry syrup

Colds, the flu, coughs, and sore throats all benefit greatly from this syrup. Additionally, it can be used during the winter to strengthen the immune system. Elderflower syrup is rich in vitamins A and C and antioxidants, and has antibacterial and antiviral properties.

Fresh elder (Sambucus canadensis or S. nigra) berry

Raw honey

Grain alcohol or 100-proof vodka (optional)

1. Harvest elderberries when they are nearly black or dark purple. Be sure to collect black elderberries (*Sambucus canadensis* or *S. nigra*) rather than red ones (*Sambucus racemosa*), which can be poisonous.

2. Place the berries in a colander and rinse well.

3. Put the washed berries in a big pot and fill it with enough water to cover them by a few inches.

4. Heat the water and berries until the water boils, then mash the berries.

5. Simmer the berries for a minimum of one hour.

6. If the mixture starts to thicken, add more water to prevent the batch from burning. Stir frequently.

7. After about an hour, let the fruit mixture boil until it has somewhat reduced in volume.

8. Then, let it cool slightly before straining it through cheesecloth or a sieve, extracting as much juice as you can.

9. While the fruit concentrate is still warm, whisk in an equal quantity of honey.

10. When stored in the refrigerator, the syrup will keep for a few months.

11. To further preserve the syrup, you can add alcohol; for every 475 ml (16 fl oz) of syrup, you need 60 ml (2 fl oz) of grain alcohol or 120 ml (4 fl oz) of 100-proof vodka.

12. Keep in the refrigerator or another cool, dry location out of direct sunlight in a glass bottle that has been disinfected.

13. 5–15 ml (1 tsp–1 tbsp) 1–3 times a day is the recommended dosage.

Elderflower glycerite

½ cup fresh elder (Sambucus nigra or S. canadensis) flowers, loosely packed (reduce to ¼ cup if using dried flowers)

Food-grade vegetable glycerine

Boiled water

1. Place elderflowers into a clean glass canning jar.

2. If using dried herbs, add enough just-boiled water to wet the herb. (This step is not necessary when using fresh herb(s) as they already contain water.) You want to be able to press the flowers with the back of a clean spoon and see a small amount of water squeeze out of them, but you don't want so much water that they're floating in it.

3. Cover the rehydrated herbs with glycerine, using just enough to cover the flowers by 1 inch.

4. Place a piece of parchment paper between the jar and the lid and seal. Label the jar, shake, and place it in a cool, dark location for 4–6 weeks, visiting every few days to give the jar a shake.

5. After the 4–6 weeks, strain the mixture through a fine-mesh sieve when time is up. It can be helpful to gently warm the jar in a water bath on the stove before straining to help thin the liquid so it passes through the strainer quickly.

6. Compost the herbs and transfer the elderflower glycerite to a clean, labelled storage bottle. Store it in a cool location and use within 1 year.

Safety considerations

No side effects or drug interactions have been reported (Hoffmann, 2003).

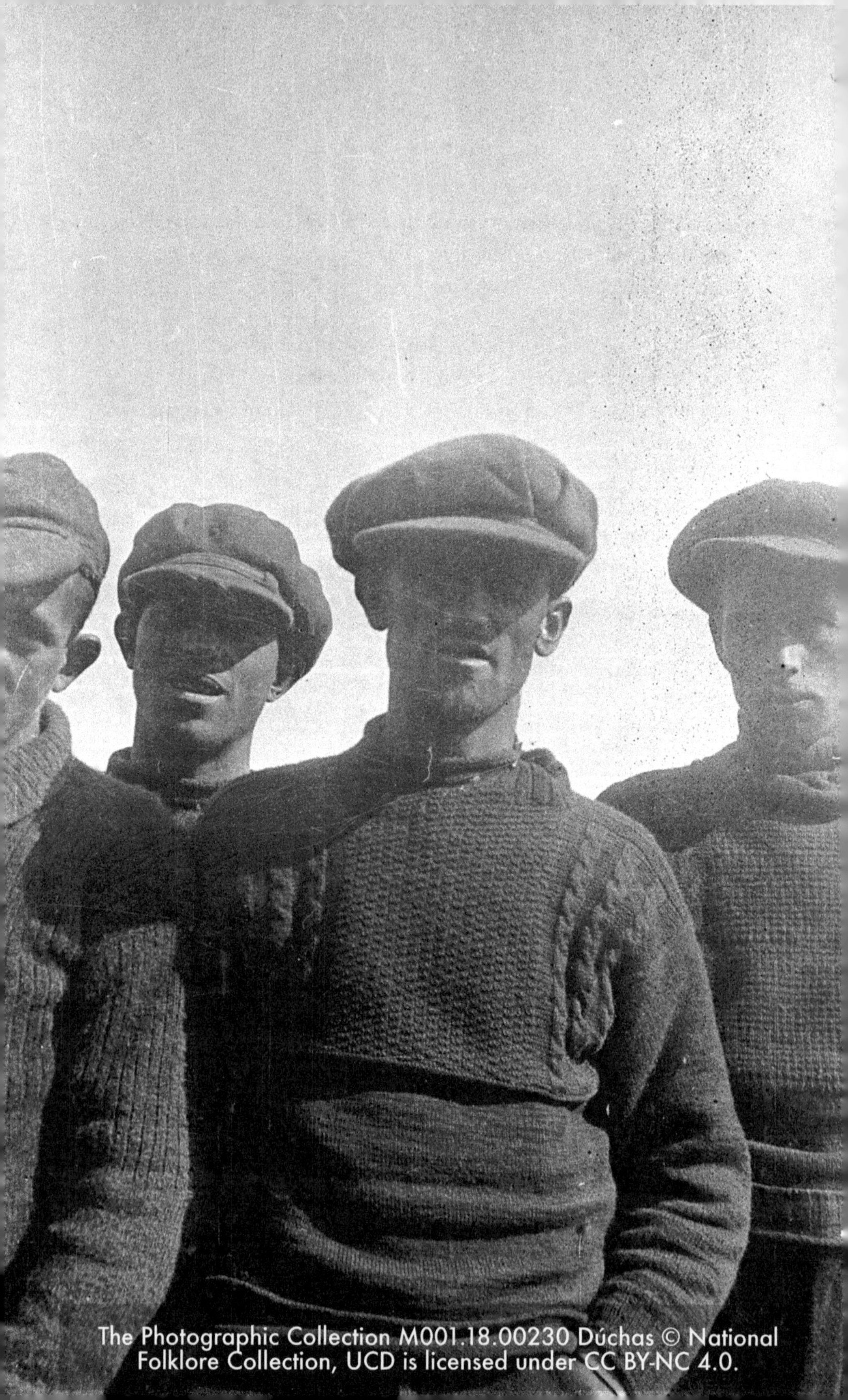

ELECAMPANE

Inula helenium

The Schools' Collection, Volume 0612, Page 0257

"Leighiseanna"
fúirthiní = ma gheibheann tú braon uisge i bpoll beag i carraig deirtear go leigheasann an t-uisge seo fáirthiní má deintear é do chimilt díobh.
Infleuenza = is cured by the maidenhairfern.
Rheumatism= is cured by ashleaves.
Insomnia = " " " | cowslips.
Sciatica pains are " " " goutwork
Epilepsy = is " " " elderleaves.
Lung troubles are " " " elecampane roots.
A Weak heart " " " casarabhán .
Bleeding - is stopped by blood grass.
Bloodpressure is cured by nettles.
Chin-cough " " " mouse-ear

> **i Another cure for the chin-cough is to let a fasting gander screech three times into your mouth.**
>
> **ii if you met a man with a white horse and ask him for a cure for the chin-cough, anything**
>
> The Schools' Collection, Volume 0612, Page 0257
>
> **Lung troubles are [cured by] elecampane.**

Elecampane has a long history of use as a tonic herb for the respiratory system. It is warming and clearing to the lower respiratory system, effectively expelling congestion and stuck energy. In addition to being an excellent expectorant, it also soothes the tissue irritation and inflammation that results from coughing.

Elecampane is helpful for treating irritating bronchial coughs, especially in children. The herb has a stimulant, expectorant effect, encouraging the coughing up of mucus from the lungs. Its warming effect on the lungs, combined with its ability to gently stimulate the clearing of mucus from the chest, makes it safe for young and old. It is particularly useful because it soothes the bronchial tube linings and is an expectorant. It can be used in almost all chest conditions and is very useful when the patient is debilitated (Gladstar, 2012).

Native American tribes used elecampane for a variety of ailments. The Cherokee used it for coughs, lung disorders, asthma, strengthening the womb, and tuberculosis. In Ayurvedic medicine, elecampane is used to clear the lungs and as a rejuvenating tonic for lung tissue. Traditional Chinese Medicine uses the flowers and leaves of two other species of elecampane (*Inula japonica* and *I. chinensis*) as a mildly warming expectorant remedy for chest congestion and a strengthening digestive bitter (Chevallier, 1996).

Herbalist David Hoffmann notes that elecampane's volatile oils are stimulating and encourage expectoration, while the mucilage (inulin) relaxes tissues and soothes discomfort (Hoffmann, 2003). The volatile oil alantolactone is anti-inflammatory, reduces mucus production, and stimulates the immune system (Chevallier, 1996). Elecampane is both an antiseptic and potent antibiotic (Edwards, 2000). It is a mild, tonic expectorant for tuberculosis, bronchial catarrh (congestion), and chronic bronchitis. It also soothes bronchial coughs.

Elecampane's capacity to relieve congestion benefits the digestive system as well. The bitter aspects of its volatile oils promote appetite and digestion (Hoffmann, 2003) and help to relieve moist congestion and poor digestion.

Elecampane is also indicated in the case of digestive deficiency such as appetite loss, fatigue and malabsorption as it "tonifies digestive qi, promotes absorption and relieves fatigue" (Holmes, 1997).

Elecampane has been taken traditionally as a tonic herb for the digestion. It stimulates the appetite and relieves dyspepsia (Gladstar, 2012).

Elecampane is blood cleansing and can support detoxification and is indicated in the case of skin conditions such as eczema and dermatosis. It is also pain relieving for such conditions as sciatica, gout and arthritis (Holmes, 1997).

Elecampane promotes menstruation and increases hormone levels to resolve oestrogen and progesterone deficiency causing menstrual disorders and premenstrual syndrome (PMS) symptoms (Holmes, 1997).

Inulin, the starch-like carbohydrate in elecampane root, has a sweet taste and can be used as a sugar substitute for diabetics (Tierra, 2003) or to help to stabilise blood sugar levels. Inulin is a prebiotic that acts as a food source for healthy gut bacteria (Nowak et al., 2012).

Elecampane specifically treats irritated bronchial coughs, especially in children. It has been used to treat bronchitis or emphysema, and also tuberculosis; it may aid with asthmatic conditions. The mucilage has a calming effect and the essential oils stimulate. As such, elecampane may help to calm inflammation and encourage expectoration. These actions are combined with an overall antibacterial effect. Its bitter principle stimulates digestion and appetite (Hoffmann, 2003).

Elecampane recipes

Lung congestion formula

Hyssop (*Hyssopus officinalis*) aerial parts (lung tonic and expectorant)

Mullein (*Verbascum thapsus*) leaf (lung tonic)

Elecampane *(Inula helenium*) root (expectorant)

1. Mix equal parts of each herb.
2. Place your herbs directly into your cafetière or infuser. Pour hot water over herbs.
3. Cover the cafetiere, mug or teapot immediately with a lid or saucer. This traps the steam and prevents the medicinal essential oils from evaporating.
4. Let the mixture steep undisturbed for 10 to 15 minutes.
5. Remove the infuser or strain the liquid into your cup. Drink it plain, or add honey and lemon to taste.

Safety considerations

Elecampane may cause allergic reactions for people with allergies to the Asteraceae family (Hoffmann, 2003). Elecampane can be irritating to mucous membranes (American Botanical Council, 1999). Large amounts of the herb may cause vomiting, diarrhoea, cramps and symptoms of paralysis (American Botanical Council, 1999).

EYEBRIGHT

Euphrasia officinalis

The Schools' Collection, Volume 0050, Page 0401

Cumphery is a cure for sprains.

Alli Compagne is a cure for blood mourn on cattle and stomach trouble.

Water-cress is a cure for liver trouble

Drowning leaf is a cure for burns

Green-Broom is a cure for kidney trouble and a pain in the back.

Dandelion cures lung disease and kidney trouble and is also good for young turkeys

Dock-leaf takes away the pain of a nettle sting.

Hemlock is a cure for Rheumatism, headache and indigestion.

Ivy cures scum in a horse's eye and is also used to remove stains.

Bog onion is used to cure a pain in the back.

Gladan is a cure for mumps.

Tansey is used to purify the blood and for killing moths.

Fox grass is used for killing worms in cattle

Nettles are used for curing warts and is also good for ducklings
Eye-bright is useful in affections of the eyes
Mostly all of the above are ready when boiling water is poured on them.

Eye infections

The Schools' Collection, Volume 0050, Page 0401

Eye-bright is useful in infections of the eyes.

Eyebright's traditional uses include allergic rhinitis, post-nasal drip, sinus headaches, sinusitis, otitis media, and red, itchy eyes associated with hay fever, and coughs and sore throats, as well as topical use of homeopathic preparations for eye fatigue and conjunctivitis (Kuhn & Winston, 2008).

Eyebright grows in meadows and common pastures, flowering in Ireland in July and August. It is good for all disorders of the eyes, the juice being mixed with white wine or distilled water and dropped into the eyes (Scott, 1986).

A lotion of eyebright made with the herb goldenseal is considered very effective against disorders of the eyes. When the eyes are very painful a warm, though not hot infusion is used; otherwise the remedy is applied cold (Scallan, 1994).

Eyebright has been described by herbalist Sara Katz (2000), in her chapter in *Planting The Future,* as having a "mild stimulating and astringent action that constricts the blood vessels of the nasal passages and the conjunctival (lachrymal) mucous membranes, helping dispel mucus and other exudates that result from inflammation" (p. 102), and further describes it as best for wet or congested conditions as opposed to dry (Katz, 2000).

Eyebright may assist with mucous membrane problems. It is useful for a variety of ailments owing to its astringent and anti-inflammatory qualities. The herb's most well-known application is in treating eye disorders including oversensitivity to light, stinging and weeping eyes, and acute or chronic inflammations. It has also been used as a compress when treating blepharitis and conjunctivitis (Hoffmann, 2003).

Eyebright - other uses

As an anticatarrhal, eyebright can be used to treat sinusitis, nasal catarrh and other congestive conditions.

Tannin and volatile oil content may contribute to the antimicrobial action of eyebright.

Peripheral uses historic claims of use for vertigo, epilepsy ear pain and dizziness.

Eyebright recipes

Eyebright eye wash and compress

Sara Katz (2000) describes using very well-strained tea of eyebright as an eyewash or compress and in other first aid applications. The suggested ratio is 1 tsp dried eyebright to 3 tsp fresh per cup of distilled water, steeped for half an hour and scrupulously strained through clean fine cloth or paper, using sterile containers. Use as an eyewash should be strained, cooled infusion, in 5–10 minute periods, repeated three times. A compress of the freshly brewed tea on sterile gauze over closed eyes can be applied for 10 to 20 minutes (Katz, 2000).

Safety considerations

No side effects or drug interactions have been reported (Hoffmann, 2003).

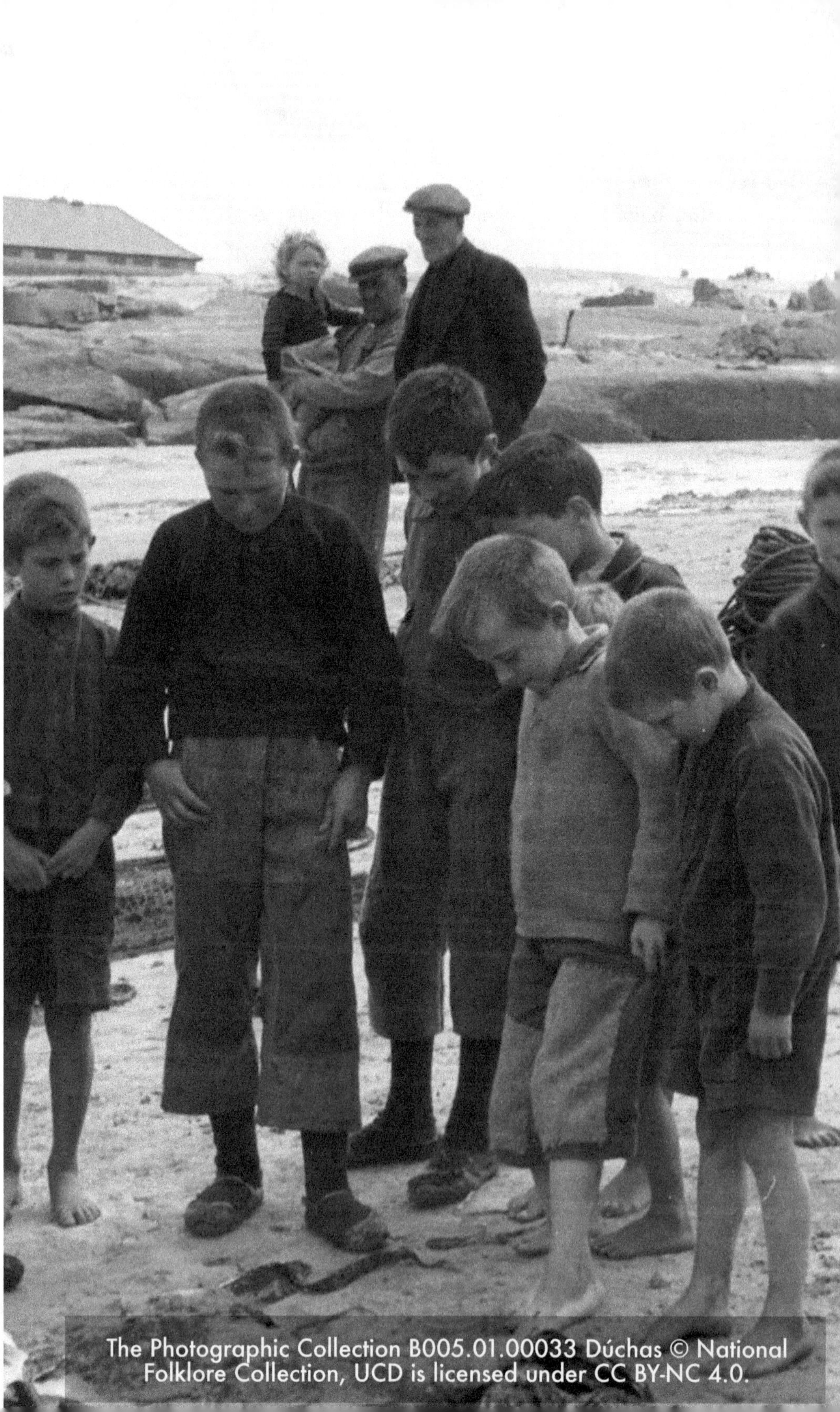

GARLIC

Allium sativum

The Schools' Collection, Volume 0021, Page 0248

Herbs are weeds that grow in fields and gardens. Some of these herbs can cure diseases but others of them are poisonous. God made them I am sure for some purpose.
Here are some of the herbs which can cure diseases. The Garlic or "on Garlóg" was an herb which grew in every garden long ago. It was said that it could cure "Mumps" or swelling around the ...

The Schools' Collection, Volume 0028, Page 0271

There are many kinds of herbs. Nettles and thistles are harmful weeds. Clover, ribgrass are found in good land. Rushes and blackheads are fond in poor land. Herbs are used for many things such as curing, dyeing. Garlic is a cure for boils. Company root is a cure for breaks and sprains. Gladam and parabaun is a cure for swelling. Dockleaf is a cure for a nettle sting. Aulder is used for dyeing. Hemlock is good for washing sheep to keep them free from insects.

The Schools' Collection, Volume 0046, Page 0197

A cure for warts is to rub the juice of a dandelion of them.
A cure for the whooping cough is to take ferret's leavings seven times after one another.
Dock leaves boiled and eaten in spring purifies the blood.
The garlic is a cure for ring worm and boils. The camomile is a cure for rheumatism. To rub a snail of a wart and then to hang the snail up on a gooseberry will the wart.

The Schools' Collection, Volume 0047, Page 0068

Garlic is a small green plant with the bulbous root. The plant is pulled and the tops are cut off.
Two or three garlic roots are then chopped up and put it into a bottle. The bottle is then filled with whiskey and is buried in the clay for nine days. The people use it for a cold or for the whooping cough.

The Schools' Collection, Volume 0050, Page 0458

Tradition tell us that the people of older times were much healthier than the people are nowadays. The only cure they had for any illness they might have were herbs.
The sowed those herbs in gardens, the same as we would sow vegetables now, but the bog-onion grew in bogs, or the banks of some rivers, or streams.

The Schools' Collection, Volume 0050, Page 0459

The garlic is a bulbous plant of the onion tribe. It's root is pounded into a mash and mixed with lard. It is used as an ointment for sore or tender feet. About half a teaspoonful of this ointment is given on milk to children for the chin-cough.

The Schools' Collection, Volume 0077, Page 0064

There are not as many cures now as there were long ago.
My Grandmother told me a few.

(1) Nettles are very good to eat during the month of March, and it is said that you should boil them and eat them three times during the month, and the person that does this will not get any disease during the year.
(2) The roots of docket leaves boiled in milk are used to cure a sick stomach.
(3) Garlic boiled in milk is good for a cold, and to put some into your shoes would cure rheumatism.

Coughs and Colds

The Schools' Collection, Volume 0047, Page 0068

Garlic is a small green plant with the bulbous root. The plant is pulled and the tops are cut off.
Two or three garlic roots are then chopped up and put it into a bottle. The bottle is then filled with whiskey and is buried in the clay for nine days. The people use it for a cold or for the whooping cough.

The Schools' Collection, Volume 0050, Page 0459

The garlic is a bulbous plant of the onion tribe. It's root is pounded into a mash and mixed with lard. It is used as an ointment for sore or tender feet. About half a teaspoonful of this ointment is given on milk to children for the chin-cough.

The Schools' Collection, Volume 0077, Page 0064

There are not as many cures now as there were long ago. My Grandmother told me a few.
(3) Garlic boiled in milk is good for a cold, and to put some into your shoes would cure rheumatism.

Garlic can bring relief from the initial stages of a cold or flu. Garlic has significant antimicrobial properties against bacteria, viruses, protozoa, worms, yeast and fungi, and it contains 18 recognised antiviral and antibacterial compounds (Gladstar, 1993).

Garlic is especially beneficial for respiratory illnesses such as bronchitis, catarrh, colds, flu and whooping cough because its volatile oils are expelled through the lungs and have antibacterial properties (Hoffmann, 2003). As an expectorant, it aids in the thinning and the body's removal of clogged phlegm from airways.

Mumps

The Schools' Collection, Volume 0021, Page 0248

The Garlic or "on Garlóg" was an herb which grew in every garden long ago. It was said that it could cure "Mumps" or swelling around the neck.

Supplementation with garlic lowers circulating markers of oxidative stress and inflammation.

Ringworm and Boils

The Schools' Collection, Volume 0046, Page 0197

The garlic is a cure for ring worm and boils.

The Schools' Collection, Volume 0028, Page 0271

Garlic is a cure for boils.

Garlic is an effective antimicrobial, acting on viruses, parasites and bacteria of the alimentary tract. It has been used externally for the treatment of the fungal infection ringworm and as a suppository against pinworm (*Enterobius vermicularis*) (Hoffmann, 2003).

Garlic – other uses

Cholesterol and cardiovascular health

Supplementation with garlic can also reduce total cholesterol levels, particularly in people with cardiovascular disease and improve other aspects of cardiovascular health (Hoffmann, 2003).

Garlic has a range of effects upon cardiovascular health. It reduces serum cholesterol and triglyceride levels while raising levels of high-density lipoproteins (HDL). It can also act as an effective inhibitor of platelet-activating factor (PAF). The hardening of arteries brought on by aging and other lifestyle decisions, such as smoking and drinking, is known as atherosclerosis. The above properties of garlic along with garlic's antioxidant properties may help in the prevention of atherosclerosis, thrombosis, hypertension, heart attack and stroke (Hoffmann, 2003).

Many studies have also been done on the ability of garlic to lower serum cholesterol levels. Human and animal (rat) studies have shown that daily garlic consumption (equivalent to 1–2 cloves of garlic a day) not only lowers serum cholesterol and triglyceride levels (Stevinson et al., 2000), but it also increases the levels of high-density lipoproteins (HDL), also known as the "good cholesterol" (Hoffmann, 2003).

This suggests that garlic may enhance liver function, which is important for regulating the body's normal levels of triglycerides and cholesterol (Horton, 2002).

The arteries harden owing to an increase of cholesterol plaque and natural calcification of the blood vessels over time. This leads to a lack of elasticity in the blood vessels, causing high blood pressure and raising risk factors of thrombosis (blood clots), impotence, heart attack and stroke. Studies have been done with garlic alone (Orekhov & Grunwald, 1997) and with statins (Budoff, 2006) and both have shown that garlic may have a positive effect on halting, and sometimes even reversing, arteriosclerosis.

Reducing blood pressure

Many studies support the use of garlic in reducing blood pressure (Reinhart, 2008), which corresponds to the idea that garlic reduces tension in the cardiovascular system and allows blood to be pumped through the body more effectively. Garlic contains aromatic chemicals that, like many other aromatics, dilate blood vessels and expand and calm circulation.

Studies show improvements when the equivalent of one clove of garlic is used daily for at least 4–6 weeks, which indicates that garlic as a part of the daily diet can support healthy blood pressure (Silagy, 1994).

Anti-clotting effects

Garlic has been shown in large doses to have anti-clotting effects in the blood (Bordia et al., 1998). Two weeks before and after surgery, garlic should be avoided in medicinal doses by those on blood-thinning drugs.

Digestion

In the digestive system, garlic sparks the digestive fire and brings heat and vitality to the digestive process. This can be aggravating to people with a warm constitution. Garlic has been shown to be effective against the bacterium *Heliobacter pylori* in conjunction with antibiotics, improving the treatment protocol by over 30% over antibiotic use alone (Tilgner, 2009). *H. pylori* has been shown to cause stomach ulcers and is implicated in certain types of stomach cancers, indicating that garlic might be effective at preventing certain digestive cancers (Hoffmann, 2003).

Garlic can generally be used as a preventative against the majority of respiratory and stomach infections. In the digestive tract, garlic is thought to kill pathogenic organisms while supporting the development of the natural bacterial flora.

Garlic recipes

Wild herb pesto

1 cup olive oil

3 cloves garlic (*Allium sativum*)

½ cup pine nuts, cashews or walnuts

Parmesan cheese, freshly grated

Assorted wild herbs

1. Have your assorted herbs chopped. Add small amounts at a time. Place enough in the blender to make a thick, green paste.

2. Place 1 cup of olive oil in the blender with 3 cloves more or less of garlic, and ½ cup of pine nuts, cashews or walnuts. Blend until very smooth.

3. Scoop into a bowl and add about ¼ cup grated parmesan cheese. Store in the refrigerator.

Garlic honey

Both garlic and honey are highly antiseptic. This combination can be used topically as an emollient antimicrobial, or spread on toast to support the immune system during a cold or the flu.

6 garlic (*Allium sativum*) cloves

85g (3 oz) raw honey

1. Use a knife to chop or a fine grater to grate raw garlic into a small bowl.

2. Add honey to garlic and mix.

3. Store in a sealed clean, glass jar for up to 3 months.

4. For internal use, take 15 ml (1 tbsp) twice a day during active infection.

5. For topical application, apply directly to wound and cover with a clean bandage at least twice a day. Optional: For increased potency in topical use only, stir in up to 2 drops of any of the following essential oils per teaspoon of honey: thyme (*Thymus vulgaris*), rosemary (*Salvia rosmarinus*), or tea tree (*Melaleuca alternifolia*).

Spicy burdock and dandelion kimchi

12 oz fresh burdock (*Arctium lappa*) root, sliced

12 oz daikon radish, chopped

12 oz fresh dandelion (*Taraxacum officinale*) leaves, chopped

2 tbsp salt

2 tbsp fresh ginger (*Zingiber officinale*) root, grated

4 garlic cloves, minced

1 cup wild chives, chopped into 2-inch pieces

1 medium carrot, cut into thin matchsticks (about 1 cup)

½ cup Korean pepper flakes

2 tbsp red miso or doenjang (Korean fermented soybean paste)

1 tbsp honey or maple syrup or agave

½ cup water

1. Peel burdock root, cut it into lengths that will fit into a bowl, and cover with water.

2. Soaking the root keeps it from oxidising and turning brown while also removing some of its bitterness.

3. While the burdock roots are soaking, you can begin to slice them diagonally into oblong pieces. The chopping of the ingredients increases the surface area to ensure thorough penetration of the brine into the thicker parts of the roots, fruits, and vegetables that will be fermenting. After you chop the roots, return them to the water to continue soaking. When all of the burdock is chopped, set the bowl aside and let it soak.

4. Chop the daikon radish into ½-inch disks.

5. Cut the dandelion leaves into 2-inch pieces.

6. In a medium-sized bowl, combine the daikon and dandelion with the salt and set aside to wilt for about 20 minutes.

7. Change the water the burdock root has been soaking in, and set aside to continue soaking. In a medium-sized bowl mix together the honey, pepper flakes and fermented soybean paste.

8. Peel and grate the ginger, and peel and mince the garlic. Chop the carrot into matchstick-sized pieces and the chives into 2-inch long sections. Combine these ingredients with the pepper paste mixture. Add a couple of tablespoons of water or so to thin the paste so it easily coats the remaining ingredients.

9. Check the radish and dandelion. They should be flexible and have exuded a fair amount of liquid. Strain off the liquid.

10. Strain the burdock root well and combine together with radish and dandelion. Taste for saltiness. If your mixture tastes overly salty, rinse and strain these ingredients before moving on to the next step.

11. Add the pepper mixture to the above ingredients and mix well, making sure there are no clumps and that all of the leaves and roots are equally coated. If using hands to combine the mixtures, wear disposable gloves to protect your skin from the spice.

Garlic and rosemary infused oil

4–8 fl oz (120–240 ml) extra virgin olive oil

5 4-inch sprigs fresh rosemary (*Salvia rosmarinus*) leaf, chopped

7 garlic (*Allium sativum*) cloves, minced

1. Chop fresh herbs and add to a dry, sanitised heat-safe glass jar.
2. Measure oil and pour over the herbs.
3. Place a cloth on the bottom of a slow cooker or saucepan, then set the glass jar on top of the cloth. Fill the vessel with enough water to the level of the mixture inside the jar.
4. Leave the lid off the jar to allow any water that might remain in the plant material to evaporate without splashing any water into the jar.
5. Set the slow cooker to warm or the stovetop to low heat, the goal being to maintain the water temperature at 180° F (82° C). Let this macerate for 4 hours, checking the temperature of the oil regularly to ensure it does not get too hot.
6. Replenish the water level in the slow cooker or saucepan with hot water as needed.
7. After four hours carefully remove the jar from the slow cooker or saucepan and set it aside to cool completely.
8. Place a cheesecloth-lined strainer inside a large dry, sanitised bowl or measuring cup with a spout. Pour the contents from the jar into the strainer. With clean, dry hands, gather the ends of the cheesecloth together and squeeze the remaining oil from the herb into the bowl.
9. Pour the oil into a dry, sanitised glass bottle or jar. Cap tightly and label.
10. Store in the refrigerator and use immediately or within 2–3 days.

Earache oil

Garlic and mullein flower are used in these antimicrobial and anti-inflammatory ear drops to soothe pain and ward off microbes, easing the ache.

<u>For the fresh garlic oil:</u>

1 part fresh garlic (*Allium sativum*) clove, finely diced

2 parts olive oil

1. Finely dice fresh garlic and add to a dry, sanitised heat-safe glass jar. Measure olive oil and pour over the garlic. Leave to infuse for 10 minutes.

2. Place a cloth at the bottom of a slow cooker or saucepan and set the glass jar on top of the cloth. Fill the vessel with enough water to cover to the level of the mixture inside the jar. Leave the lid off the jar to allow water in the garlic to evaporate.

3. Set the slow cooker to warm or the stovetop to low heat, the goal being to maintain the water temperature at 120–140° F (49–60° C). Let this macerate for 4 hours, checking the temperature of the oil regularly to ensure it doesn't get too hot.

4. Replenish the water level in the slow cooker or saucepan with hot water as needed.

5. After four hours carefully remove the jar from the slow cooker or saucepan and set it aside to cool completely.

6. Place a cheesecloth-lined strainer inside a large dry, sanitised bowl or measuring jug. Pour the contents from the jar into the strainer. With

clean, dry hands, gather the ends of the cheesecloth together and squeeze the remaining oil from the herb into the bowl.

7. Pour the oil into a dry, sanitised glass jar, cap, and let it settle overnight.

8. Strain the oil again, being careful to avoid pouring out any of the remaining herb particulates that have settled to the bottom of the jar.

9. Pour the garlic infused oil into a dry, sanitized glass bottle or jar. Cap tightly and label.

<u>For the earache oil:</u>

1 part fresh garlic (*Allium sativum*) clove infused oil

1 part fresh mullein (*Verbascum thapsus*) flower infused oil (page 148)

1. Measure the appropriate amount of each herbal oil and transfer both to a dark-coloured, sanitised, dry glass container.

2. Cover and shake well to combine.

3. Label, and store in a cool, dark place for up to 1 year.

4. To use, place 1–3 drops of room temperature oil in achy ears 3–4 times daily. Do not use if the eardrum is perforated.

Safety considerations

At high doses, garlic may irritate the intestinal mucosa, causing nausea, diarrhoea, vomiting and burning of the mouth. However, in humans, daily administration of high doses of garlic essential oil (approximately 120mg, equivalent to 60g/day fresh garlic) over a period of 3 months did not cause any adverse effects. Contact dermatitis from occupational exposure has been reported (Hoffmann, 2003).

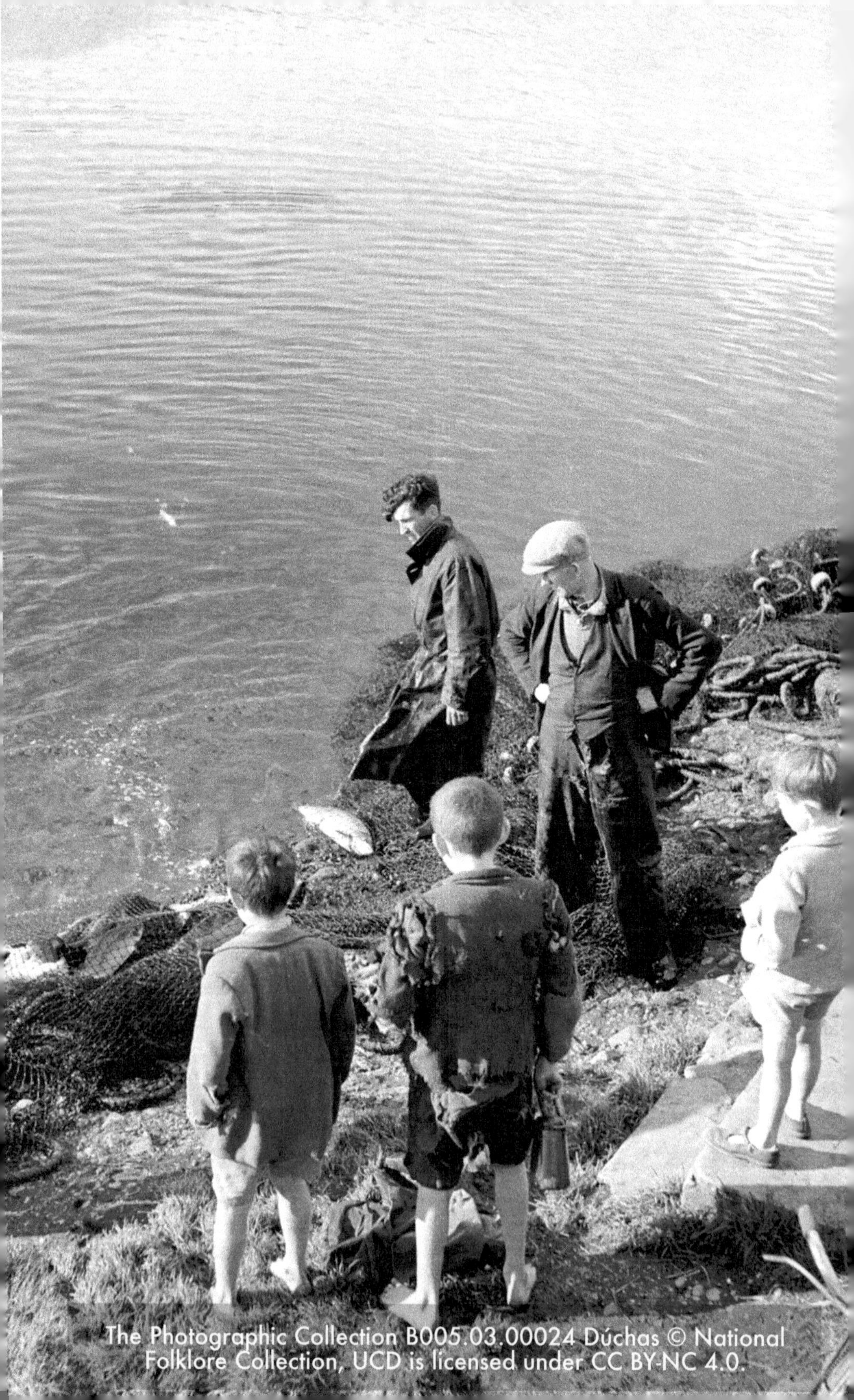

GERANIUM

Geranium maculatum (Cranesbill)

The Schools' Collection, Volume 0687, Page 0424

The most common and harmful weeds growing in our district are, thistles, nettles, scutch grass, bulky shanks, hemlock, chicken weed and grounsel.
Rushes grow on bad land, and clover and bulky shanks called buacallán in Irish grow on good land.
Dandelions are very good to eat and some people eat them.
The milk of the dandelion is good for warts.
Iodine is made out of seaweed.
Crane's Bill is a little pink flower with flat leaves and it cures Rheumatism. Every bit of it is boiled except the roots, and sugar is put into it. Then it is drank and the Rheumatism is cured.
Dock leaves cures nettle stings by putting the leaves to the sting and keeping [them there until the sting is gone.]

The Schools' Collection, Volume 0406, Page 0572

Dandelion is used for all kinds of stomach trouble. It is prepared like tea and drunk either hot or cold just as Cranes Bill is. It is a great thing for a bad stomach.

The Schools' Collection, Volume 0689, Page 0261

"Groundsil" and "scutch" are the most harmful weeds growing in the garden because they spread rapidly.
The "wart weed" is an herb with a tiny yellow flower. If one breaks the stem a milky fluid comes out which if rubbed to the wart will cure it.
The "mouse ear" is an herb which has a leaf shaped like a mouse's ear. This herb cures the "burst".
If one drinks the water of boiled "cranes bill" it will cure back-ache.
"Foxtongue" gets it's name because it is shaped like a fox's [tongue]

The Schools' Collection, Volume 0704, Page 0297

There was a man in Drewstown who had the cure for kidney trouble. He would get herbs called "Early Spring" and "Cranes bill". He would boil them and mix them with new milk and then give the drink to the complaining person. This is a reliable cure.

The Schools' Collection, Volume 0546, Page 0127

There were different herbs used for curing different ailments. The Wartweed was used to cure warts. Robin Run the Hedge is a cure for biles and carbuncles. This is a sticky weed with small green berries attached to it. It grows in a creeping manner along hedges. Rib grass is a cure for ringworms. Cranes Bill is a cure for tetters. It is found in ditches.

The Schools' Collection, Volume 0738, Page 0198

There is a weed called the Cranes Bill which is a cure for pains when it is boiled in milk. The Cranes Bill blossoms a little red flower and it is usually found in hedges.

The most harmful weeds growing on the farms in this district are lambs quarter, scutch grass pressure and many others. If these weeds were not kept in check by weeding they would ruin all our crops. Old people can use many kinds of weeds to cure different diseases but the practise has nearly died out.
There is a cure for a corn from the dandelion, squeeze the shank of the dandelion on to the corn and it will fall out.
There is a cure for the sting of a knettle [nettle], get a docking and rub the sting with it and it will be cured. There is a cure for warts, get a raw potatoe and rub it to the wart twice a day and it will be cured. There is also a cure for a cold, get the roots of garlic and boil it in new-milk and drink it very hot.
There is a weed which grows in the hedges and it is called robin run the hedge. There are little round things on this weed which would stick to your clothes if you went near them. Thistles are harmful weeds because they spread [quickly if not cut]

The Schools' Collection, Volume 0923, Page 0059

In olden times people used every herb as a cure to some ailment. They used "Cranes Bill" to make medicine which was good for Consumption. "Fellons" grass was good for Fellons or a rash on the hands. "Comfrey" was used to cure a sprain. The old people used Camanmile to make medicine which wass good for a cough. They used "house-leek" for sore eyes. With "Ladies Mantle" they used to stop blood. The old people can point out these herbs in the fields and they had small plots in which they used to plant such things.

The Schools' Collection, Volume 0687, Page 0424

Crane's Bill is a little pink flower with flat leaves and it cures Rheumatism. Every bit of it is boiled except the roots, and sugar is put into it. Then it is drank and the Rheumatism is cured.

The Schools' Collection, Volume 0406, Page 0572

Dandelion is used for all kinds of stomach trouble. It is prepared like tea and drunk either hot or cold just as Cranes Bill is. It is a great thing for a bad stomach.

The Schools' Collection, Volume 0689, Page 0261

If one drinks the water of boiled "cranes bill" it will cure back-ache.

The Schools' Collection, Volume 0704, Page 0297

There was a man in Drewstown who had the cure for kidney trouble. He would get herbs called "Early Spring" and "Cranes bill". He would boil them and mix them with new milk and then give the drink to the complaining person. This is a reliable cure.

The Schools' Collection, Volume 0546, Page 0127

Cranes Bill is a cure for tetters. It is found in ditches.

The Schools' Collection, Volume 0738, Page 0198

There is a weed called the Cranes Bill which is a cure for pains when it is boiled in milk. The Cranes Bill blossoms a little red flower and it is usually found in hedges.

The Schools' Collection, Volume 0923, Page 0059

In olden times people used every herb as a cure to some ailment. They used "Cranes Bill" to make medicine which was good for Consumption.

American cranesbill (Geranium) is an effective astringent historically used for diarrhoea, dysentery and haemorrhoids. It is also indicated for the treatment of menorrhagia (excessive blood loss during menstruation) (Hoffmann, 2003)

Safety considerations

No side effects or drug interactions have been reported.

GOLDENROD

Solidago spp.

The Schools' Collection, Volume 0692, Page 0258

John McCormack, (40) Newcastle. Local Cures Mary McCormack

Long ago people cured their ailments with certain herbs such as the Golden Rod, Sun Dew, Dog Daisy leaves, Mouse's Ear, Dandelion, Docks, Crowfoot, Chickenweed, Heart Herb, Blood-Weed, Gooseberry Thorns and Ivy Leaves.

For kidney trouble they used the Golden Rod. They boiled it in new milk and drank the juice.

For a heavy cold they used the Dog Daisy boiled with the Dandelion in water.

The dock eased the sting of a nettle by rubbing it to where the sting was.

For a cut finger or anything that began to bleed, they pressed the blood-weed against it saying "In the name of the Father and of the Son and of the Holy-Ghost". After a while the blood stopped.

> **For a swelling on the foot or on the hands they made a poultice of crow-foot and chickenweed and applied it as hot as possible.**
> **For a bad heart they used the Heart herb. They boiled it with Mouse's Ear or Sun Dew and made a warm drink.**
> **The gooseberry thorns were used for a sty.**
>
> The Schools' Collection, Volume 0692, Page 0258
>
> **For kidney trouble they used the Golden Rod. They boiled it in new milk and drank the juice.**

One of the herbal uses of goldenrod is related to its toning, antimicrobial, anti-inflammatory and diuretic effects upon the urinary system. The use of various goldenrod species for urinary tract support is seen in some Native American traditions. Cherokee herbalist and author J.T. Garrett (2003) describes the use of *Solidago odora* as a diuretic for addressing kidney stones and oedema, and the Lumbee have traditionally made a tea with the flowers of *S. canadensis* for a variety of bladder and kidney issues (Boughman & Oxendine, 2003).

Culpeper (1995) writes of the plant's profound diuretic effects to "... provoke urine in abundance..." (p. 120) in order to ease the passing of kidney stones in the bladder and kidneys.

Goldenrod has been used for upper respiratory catarrh, whether it be acute or chronic. Additionally, the plant can be used to treat influenza in conjunction with other herbs.

Its carminative properties point to a role in the treatment of flatulent dyspepsia. As an anti-inflammatory urinary tract antiseptic, goldenrod may be helpful in cystitis, urethritis and similar conditions affecting this system. As a gargle, goldenrod can be effective for laryngitis and pharyngitis. It may be applied externally to promote the healing of wounds.

Goldenrod recipes

Formula for acute allergies with sinus congestion

Liquorice (*Glycyrrhiza glabra*) root

Goldenrod (*Solidago* spp.) aerial parts

Horseradish (*Armoracia rusticana*) root

1. Mix equal parts of each herb.
2. Place your herbs directly into your cafetière or infuser. Pour hot water over herbs.
3. Cover the cafetière, mug or teapot immediately with a lid or saucer. This traps the steam and prevents the medicinal essential oils from evaporating.
4. Let the mixture steep undisturbed for 10 to 15 minutes.
5. Remove the infuser or strain the liquid into your cup. Drink it plain, or add honey and lemon to taste.

Safety considerations

People sensitive to plants in the Asteraceae family may have an allergic reaction to goldenrod (Hoffmann, 2003).

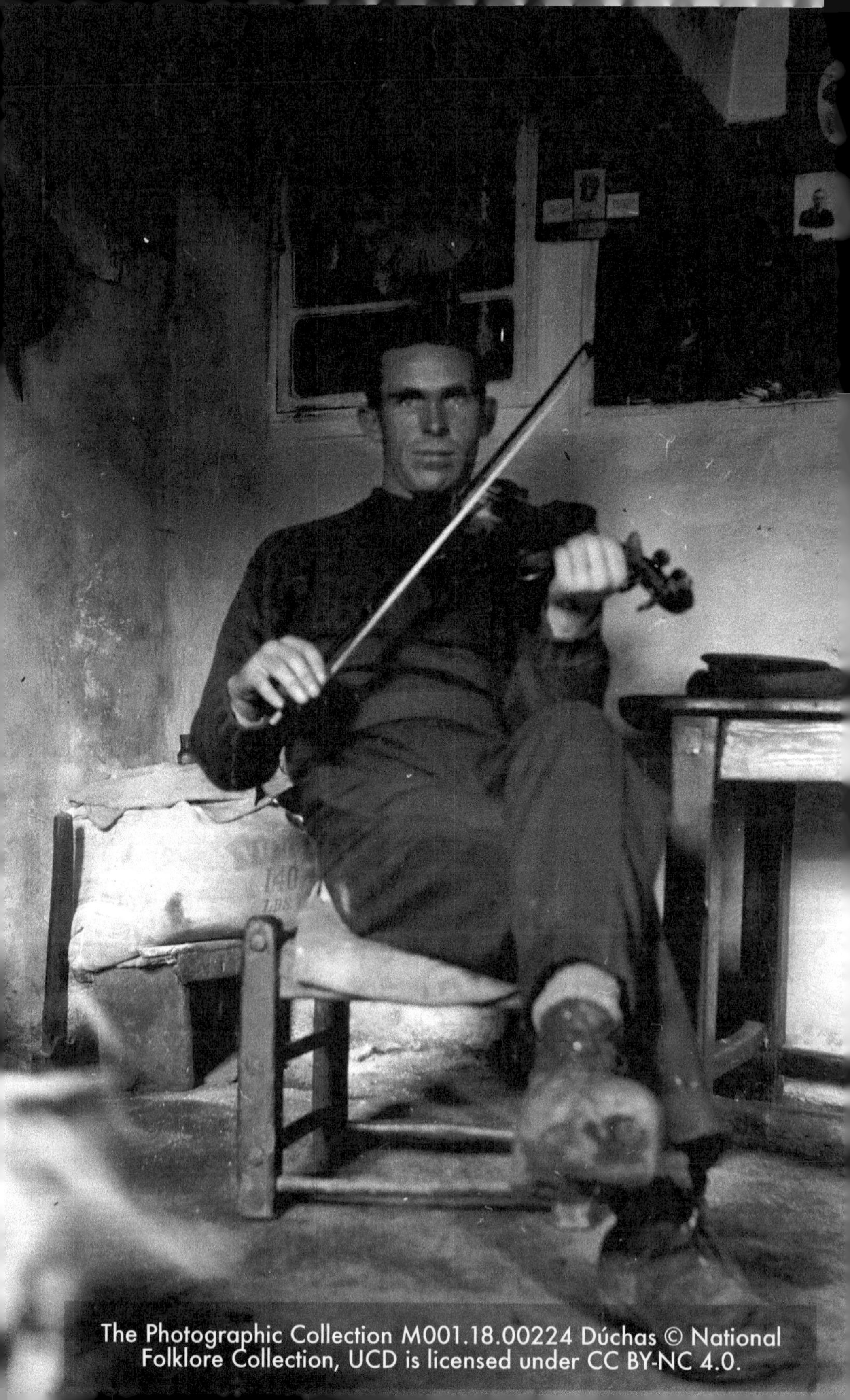

HORE HOUND

Marrubium vulgare

The Schools' Collection, Volume 0527, Page 0047

White horehound is found in waste ground. The whole plant is aromatic and bitter, and is a common remedy here for coughs.

The Schools' Collection, Volume 0690, Page 0013

Toothache:- The cure of a toothache is when people are making a grave, if you get a tooth, put it in your mouth and keep it in it till you say one Hail Mary.
Ringworm:- The cure of ringworn is to get a gold ring and put it over the ringworm three times and make the sign of the Cross
Sore Eye:- The cure of a stye on your eye is to go into the garden and get ten gooseberry thorns and point nine of them towards your eye and make the Sign of the Cross with each one and throw away the tenth one across your shoulder.
Cold:- If you gather a branch of the common Horehound herb, and boil it for one hour in a quart of water, strained and mixed with liquorice ball and sugar, and it will cure any cold.

Warts:- To cure warts put a snail on the wart and then put him on a stalk of a hawthorn, and when the snail withers the wart will go too.
Rheumatism:- To cure rheumatism carry a small potato in your pocket and when it withers put in a fresh one.

The Schools' Collection, Volume 0662, Page 0097

Horehound tea is still used in the district as a cure for a cold, but as Mr Michael Caffrey of Crumlin say it is very bad-tasted, and hence not as popular as the ordinary tea. He grows Horehound in his garden

The Schools' Collection, Volume 0675, Page 0136

Boxty Bread was made from oaten meal baked on a griddle. I think it must be over 70 years since it was made in this village.
Horehound Tea was used here abut 70 years ago. The horehound flower is a blue flower. Long ago the flower heads were pulled and dried in the sun. When dried it was put in canisters and then used for tea, which was very strong. Pepper and sugar were put on it but not milk.
The potato cake was made with cooked mashed potatoes, baking soda and milk. It was white and baked in a pot oven. This cake is seldom made now.
Stampy bread was made from wheaten meal. When ready for the oven marks were put on the loaf so it could be cut easily.
Brown Bread which was called "Brown John" was very large and was baked on a griddle.

There are two varieties of horehound used in Western materia medicas to be conscious of: white horehound (*Marrubium vulgare*) and black horehound (*Ballota nigra*). Although these herbs share a common name, they are predominantly used in different ways and are not analogues for one another.

White horehound is a very bitter herb in the mint family and an age-old remedy for coughs in European folk and traditional medicine.

Traditionally, white horehound was used for whooping cough and in syrup form for coughs, colds, asthma and other pulmonary issues (Hoffmann, 2003).

A warm infusion of horehound can help ease throat hoarseness, disperse heat, promote sweating and resolve mucus. The cold infusion promotes urination and helps stop sweating and excessive discharge (Holmes, 1989; Hoffmann, 2003).

Owing to its expectorant action, horehound is a valuable herb for supporting the clearance of bronchitis, particularly when there is a non-productive cough. It works by encouraging mucus production and relaxing the smooth muscles of the bronchi.

Because horehound works on both the upper and lower sections of the respiratory system, it is a profound herb to draw from for a number of bronchial complaints including non-productive coughs, wheezing, pharyngitis, sinusitis, bronchitis, asthma and tuberculosis where the catarrh is dried out and adhesive (Holmes, 1989; Wood, 2008). Horehound is commonly used in both acute and chronic congestive bronchial conditions. Given horehound's primary affinity for the respiratory system and secondary affinity for the liver, one instance where horehound would be especially indicated is in recurrent sore throat symptoms arising from chronic liver congestion (Holmes, 1989).

As Australian herbalist Dorothy Hall describes, when one feels the first tickle of a cold or cough coming on, usually in the back of the throat, horehound is indicated (Hall, 1988). As Matthew Wood (2008) observes, soreness in the throat begins to increase alongside an increase in salivation, which begins to irritate the larynx and bronchi. When these secretions dry out, a lack of appetite, digestive dryness, boggy mucus and dry, harsh coughing can occur (Wood, 2008). This is one respiratory system pattern where horehound would be indicated for use. The relaxing diaphoretic nature of horehound makes it a useful herbal aid for respiratory infections where symptoms including fever, painful swollen throat, hoarseness and sinus mucus drainage are present.

Goldenrod (*Solidago* spp.) is often formulated with horehound for sinusitis-type conditions (Holmes, 1989). Horehound also carries an analgesic action, which has been found to significantly ease pain, making it a useful herb for pain associated with coughs and sore throats. Its antispasmodic action is also useful in this regard and can help relax a painful, spastic cough in addition to relieving gas pains throughout the gastrointestinal system (de Souza et al., 1998).

Although horehound is most commonly used for its effects on the respiratory system, it can also be used to support the female reproductive system. Both traditionally and in the modern era, horehound has been drawn on to help promote menstrual flow (Cook, 1869; Storl, 2012). British herbalists have been reported to use horehound for infertility connected with excess androgen levels in the body. In excess androgenism, mucus can interfere with the descent of the egg through the fallopian tubes as well as its implantation in the uterus. As such, this application is understandable given horehound's ability to expectorate and modulate mucus levels. Matthew Wood also mentions the benefits of using horehound in his practice for "thin women who gain abdominal fat in their forties and fifties from high androgen" (Wood, 2008: 335).

Horehound also lends some support for the gastrointestinal tract. In modern herbal practice, horehound is used for loss of appetite, non-ulcer dyspepsia, gas, distention and constipation (Skenderi, 2003).

As a bitter digestive stimulant and detoxicant diuretic, horehound has been used for ages to address metabolic disorders specifically related to the liver and kidneys. The general symptom picture here would present with digestive disorders, portal congestion, headaches and acidosis among others (Holmes, 1989).

Horehound has been found in clinical practice to calm the heart and relieve heart palpitations while restoring normal glandular secretions (Tierra, 1988). In Tunisian folk medicine, horehound was used as a hypotensive and cardiotonic herb (Zarai et al., 2011). Although there are no human clinical studies published confirming these effects, animal studies have been performed suggesting horehound's antihypertensive and vasorelaxant effects, which have been observed traditionally for many years (El Bardai et al., 2003; El Bardai et al., 2004).

Horehound has been applied topically as an ointment or wash for sores, ulcers, scabs, bites and cuts (Holmes, 1989). The promotion of tissue repair is a less common application of horehound (Holmes, 1989).

Given horehound's prominent bitter flavour, it is most commonly used in a formula with other herbs to assist in balancing the taste, energetics and action (Skenderi, 2003). A few common corrigents for balancing horehound's bitterness are honey, sugar or freshly squeezed lemon or lime juice (Moore, 2003). Horehound is occasionally used as a substitute for hops (*Humulus lupulus*) when making beer – horehound ale can still be found for purchase in Europe.

When prepared as a hot infusion, its diaphoretic action will become more prominent, making it an efficient herb to help promote sweating and clear sputum. As a cold infusion, horehound's diuretic and digestive stimulant actions are more pronounced and sweating is decreased (Holmes, 1989; Moore, 2003). A popular preparation of horehound is as a syrup with honey added for an additional soothing action on the respiratory mucosa (Tierra, 1988). Note that if one exceeds the standard dosage range for using horehound, it could induce nausea and vomiting (Holmes, 1989).

White horehound is effective as a remedy for diseases of the lung. It was given to ease consumption in years gone by, and asthmatic and others with congested lungs obtain great relief from it. A decoction of the herb combined with rue, liquorice root, marshmallow root and hyssop can help with a chronic cough and even with consumption. Made into a syrup, white horehound is both a tonic and a remedy for coughs in children; it has the added benefit of settling their stomachs. An infusion is adequate for the common cold and will bring ease and a sense of well-being if taken three or four times in the day.

The leaves of white horehound can be dried, powdered and used as a vermifuge (parasite remedy) while the leaves can also be boiled with lard into an ointment useful for healing cuts and abrasions. Candied horehound made by boiling the fresh plant and extracting its juices is an easy means of administering the herb. Large doses of the herb will have a mild laxative effect. White horehound restores appetite, strengthens the heart, helps to remedy malaria and has a tonic effect on the liver (Scallan, 1994).

Black horehound (*Ballota nigra*)

Black horehound is an excellent remedy for calming nausea and vomiting when the cause lies within the nervous system, rather than in the stomach. It may be safely used for motion sickness, for example, in which nausea is triggered through the inner ear and the central nervous system. This herb is also of value in treating nausea and vomiting caused by pregnancy or nervousness. Black horehound has a reputation as a normaliser of menstrual function and as a mild expectorant.

Horehound recipes

Horehound cough drops with honey

1 cup dried organic white horehound (*Marrubium vuigare*)

2 cups water

1 cup honey

1. Add horehound and water to a small saucepan. Bring to a boil, and simmer gently for 20 minutes. The liquid should look almost like coffee.

2. Allow the liquid to cool. Squeeze out as much liquid as you can by straining it out. After discarding the horehound, return the strained liquid to the small saucepan.

3. To the horehound liquid, add honey. Simmer gently, stirring often. Drip a little drop from the spoon into a jar of ice water. When the drip turns into a very hard little boil (like a cough drop), the mixture is ready.

4. Pour liquid onto a cookie sheet, or flat sheet pan.

5. Working from the edges, scoop up teaspoonfuls of the mixture, and roll into balls. Place on parchment-lined cookie sheet, being careful not to let cough drops touch each other.

6. Work quickly before the mixture hardens.

7. When the cough drops are completely cooled (allow at least an hour), store in an airtight container in a cool, dry location.

Safety considerations

White horehound

Owing to its bitter action, it is contraindicated with kidney stones, gallbladder disease, dysmenorrhea, gastroesophageal reflux disease, hiatus hernia, gastritis and peptic ulcers (Hoffmann, 2003). Since white horehound was traditionally used as an emmenagogue herb, it is advised not to be used during pregnancy except under the strict supervision of a qualified healthcare practitioner (Gardner & McGuffin, 2013). Frequent use for extended periods of time could cause hypertension in some people, particularly the elderly with episodic hypertension (Moore, 2003).

Black horehound

No side effects or drug interactions have been reported (Hoffmann, 2003).

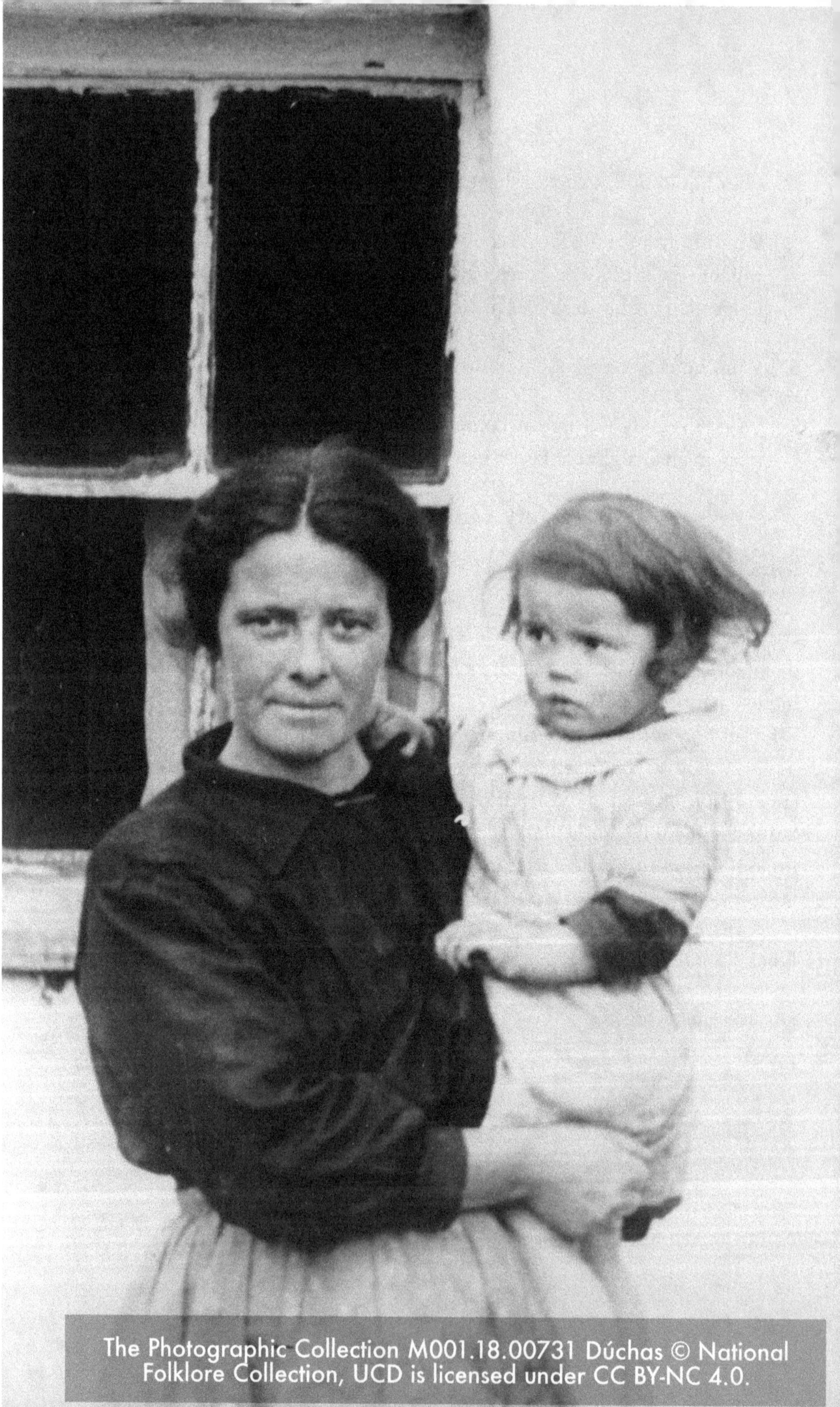

IVY

Hedera helix

The Schools' Collection, Volume 0056, Page 0151

Uses of Herbs

1. (a) Ivy-leaf cured coughs. Ivy was found growing on a wall with lime. To a pot of
ivy-leaves a half-pot of water was added. It was boiled down to half the amount. This was then strained, and liquorice, sugar-candy, and a glass of whiskey added. This was a great cure for colds.

(b) Ivy-Leaf was also a remedy for drawing water from flesh. It was put on as a bandage.

Nettles were used as a cure for Rheumatism by placing them between two sheets.

Chicken-weed for a poultice.

Allderberry made wine which was good for many ailments and diseases.

A yellow flower (which grows with a leaf like cabbage) was dried and smoked as a cure for Consumption.

Skin and burns

The Schools' Collection, Volume 0053, Page 0120

Ivy leaf is great for burns.

The Schools' Collection, Volume 0056, Page 0151

Uses of Herbs

1. (a) Ivy-leaf cured coughs. Ivy was found growing on a wall with lime. To a pot of
ivy-leaves a half-pot of water was added. It was boiled down to half the amount. This was then strained, and liquorice, sugar-candy, and a glass of whiskey added. This was a great cure for colds.

(b) Ivy-Leaf was also a remedy for drawing water from flesh. It was put on as a bandage.

The Schools' Collection, Volume 0079, Page 0354

Ivy leave, is a cure for corns.

The consumption of ivy would not be recommended today, but its historical use as a bandage is well known. Michael Scott notes in *An Irish Herbal*: "It flowers in June, with the fruit ripening in winter. The juice of the leaves cures wounds, ulcers, burns and scalds and when applied with oil of roses it cures headaches" (Scott, 1986).

Safety considerations

Ivy is harmful if eaten and is a skin irritant.

LADY'S MANTLE

Alchemilla vulgaris (syn. A. xanthochlora)

The Schools' Collection, Volume 0687, Page 0147

Cures collected from Mrs Reilly Johnstown aged 75

Wood sorrel chopped up finely mixed with lard is good for sores of every description

For Boils: Plantain leaf for boils and swellings. Take out the tough veins of the leaf and chop finely. Make some oatmeal gruel and pour over the chopped leaves. Apply as an ointment. The whole leaf is also applied to cuts.

The lady mantle: A plant which used to grow in the vicinity was an infallible cure for burns. It was chopped and mixed with unsalted butter. The blessed Virgin is supposed to have touched it sometime hence its virtue.

Leaves of the elder tree boiled in oatmeal and water was good for boils and swellings of any kind

> The Schools' Collection, Volume 0119, Page 0463
>
> The old people made use of many herbs. The leaves of Lady's Mantle boiled with unsalted butter made a liniment which was a cure for a cold in the chest. When rubbed of the chest it cured the person.
>
> Buachaill a'Tighe was an herb which was growing on every thatched house. It was growing on the roof where the side-wall and gable met. It had a thick juicy leaf. After long periods of drought it was able to live on. It conserved the water in its leaves sufficient to last it for the whole year. It was used to make an eye-water which was used for sore eyes. One boy said that Buchaill a'Tighe boiled in milk and the decoction given to the changling would bring back the child which was.

> The Schools' Collection, Volume 0687, Page 0147
>
> The lady's mantle: A plant which used to grow in the vicinity was an infallible cure for burns. It was chopped and mixed with unsalted butter. The blessed Virgin is supposed to have touched it sometime hence its virtue.

> The Schools' Collection, Volume 0119, Page 0463
>
> The old people made use of many herbs. The leaves of Lady's Mantle boiled with unsalted butter made a liniment which was a cure for a cold in the chest. When rubbed of the chest it cured the person.

In various areas of Europe, lady's mantle was relied on to aid both burns and wounds, while in Turkey, it was utilised for its vulnerary and anti-infective capabilities to address cuts (Kanak et al., 2025).

When German herbals were translated into English during the Renaissance, the plant was called lady's mantle, translated from *Frauenmantel,* so called because of the folds in the leaves that made it look like a woman's cloak. This also helped to cement its association with the

Virgin Mary, since the lobes of the leaves were thought to resemble a virgin's mantle. Once the name lady's mantle was given by Tragus in 1532 and later endorsed by Linnaeus, the herb would, from then on, be primarily associated with folk tradition and female concerns, rather than for its efficacy as a wound aid (Grieve, 1931 / 1971; Wood, 1997).

Despite this, modern *in vivo* and *in vitro* research on lady's mantle has reinforced its efficacy in wound repair in part owing to its phenolic compounds and antioxidant actions (Tasić-Kostov et al., 2019).

Lady's mantle has been widely used in folk medicine throughout Europe. It helps reduce pains associated with menstrual periods. It also has a role in easing symptoms of menopause. As an emmenagogue, it can stimulate proper menstrual flow. It is also a useful uterine astringent, helpful in menorrhagia (excessive menstrual bleeding). Its astringency makes it beneficial in the treatment of diarrhoea, as a mouthwash for sores and ulcers and as a gargle for laryngitis (Hoffmann, 2003).

Lady's mantle recipes

Astringent under-eye mask

Astringent herbs combine with eye-friendly cucumber in this mask for baggy or puffy eyes.

2 tsp lady's mantle (*Alchemilla vulgaris*) aerial parts, powder

1 tsp white cosmetic clay

2–3 tsp cucumber (*Cucumis sativus*) hydrosol

1. Combine all dry ingredients.
2. Slowly add hydrosol until you reach a mud-like consistency.
3. Apply gently to the area under the eyes.
4. Leave on for 20–30 minutes.

5. Rinse with warm water.

6. Gently pat skin.

Safety considerations

Some herbalists note that it should not be used during pregnancy (Chevallier, 2000). No side effects or drug interactions have been reported.

MARSHMALLOW

Althaea officinalis

The Schools' Collection, Volume 0057, Page 0123

People all know that they should rub the affected part with dock leaf and strange both it is remarked grow side by side. Dock is a very useful herb and it is so called from the colour of its roots which is the most valuable part of the plant. It is used for hemorrhage of the lungs. The best way of using it as a remedy is, wash roots and boil half a pound of the powdered root in a pint of golden syrup. This can then be taken in teaspoonful doses. It is also used in liver complaints and is a mild laxative.

Marshmallow is a nice herb with purple flowers and dark green leaves. The crushed roots will draw out inflammation from boils or wounds when other things fail and it is called Mortification Herb by most country people and when the leaves are brewed (like tea) it is known to cure the most obstinate cough.

Coltsfoot, a little of the dried leaves put on a plate and lighted will gradually smoulder away and the smoke inhaled

Inflammation

The Schools' Collection, Volume 0057, Page 0123

> **Marshmallow is a nice herb with purple flowers and dark green leaves. The crushed roots will draw out inflammation from boils or wounds when other things fail.**

This reference ties in with the traditional and early uses of marshmallow including its employment as a poultice for inflammation (Whelan, n.d.). Dr Ellingwood (1919) also described marshmallow as helpful for inflammation.

Marshmallow flowers may be used externally for skin inflammation, and the root is also excellent as a poultice for skin irritations. Marshmallow root releases slippery, soft mucilage when steeped in water. In fact, the entire plant "abounds with mucilage" (Grieve, 1931/1971: 507). Hoffmann notes that it may be incorporated into "drawing ointments used for abscesses and boils" (Hoffmann, 2003: 526). In traditional Persian healthcare, marshmallow extract is used to bathe babies, soothing itchy irritation and rashes (Kianitalaei et al., 2019). Herbalist Matthew Wood (2004) underscores marshmallow's widespread application in addressing diverse skin issues, ranging from dryness and roughness to dandruff and insect bites.

Marshmallow is frequently applied externally as an emollient for varicose veins and ulcers and as a component in drawing ointments for boils and abscesses.

Marshmallow – other uses

According to Priest & Priest, marshmallow is considered a soothing demulcent for inflamed and irritated states of mucous membranes. It is especially appropriate for elderly people with conditions affecting the genitourinary tract or gastrointestinal chronic inflammatory diseases. Acute respiratory disease, gastroenteritis, peptic ulcer, cystitis, urethritis, mouth and throat irritation, inflamed haemorrhoids, wounds, burns and scalds, bedsores, abscesses, boils, and skin ulcers were among the specific indications (Hoffmann, 2003).

A great demulcent, marshmallow is recommended whenever such an action is required owing to its high mucilage content. Marshmallow leaf is primarily used in the lungs and urinary system, and the root is mainly used in the digestive system. Applying marshmallow root may help with inflammatory gastrointestinal illnesses, such as colitis, peptic ulcers, throat inflammations and gastritis. The leaf may help with respiratory catarrh, bronchitis, irritating coughs, urethritis, cystitis and urinary gravel (Hoffmann, 2003).

Gastroesophageal reflux disease (GERD)

Marshmallow can help ease the symptoms of gastroesophageal reflux disease (GERD), a condition where stomach contents, including acid, flow backward into the oesophagus instead of moving forward through the digestive tract (Luchterhand, 2012). This can cause frequent heartburn, a burning sensation behind the breastbone, and may lead to damage to the oesophageal lining.

To use marshmallow for respite from symptoms, the usual dosage is 5–6 grams daily, equivalent to about 2–3 tbsp. Prepare a tea by infusing the leaves or roots in hot water, and drink 1 tbsp (or less) of the tea three times a day (Luchterhand, 2012).

Dry cough

Marshmallow, as described by herbalist Matthew Wood (2004), tends to be particularly effective in situations where dryness coincides with irritation. It demonstrates its efficacy especially in cases where the tongue presents with redness and a dry, cracked texture; its salty nature makes it useful in addressing conditions characterised by hardened tissues, as it draws in water (Wood, 2004).

Marshmallow root for dry cough, moderate stomach mucosal irritation and oral and pharyngeal mucosal irritation, as well as the marshmallow leaf for dry cough and oral/pharyngeal mucosal irritation, have been approved by the German Commission E. According to Hoffmann (2003), marshmallow has emollient, expectorant, diuretic, anti-inflammatory and demulcent properties.

When used as an infusion or decoction, marshmallow mucilage cools and coats the inflamed tissues with its gel, relieving dry, sore throats. Some herbalists believe that a cold infusion of the root is the most effective way to extract this beneficial mucilage, although Richo Cech (2000) recommends a water decoction of the dried root and a cold-water infusion of the leaves and flowers.

Respiratory complaints

Marshmallow is helpful for respiratory complaints, GI tract problems like irritable bowel syndrome (IBS) and colitis, and urinary tract discomforts. Both the root and the leaves can be used for these purposes, but Chevallier (2000) suggests the leaves for cystitis and frequent urination. Because the mucilaginous polysaccharides would not physically be able to coat the urinary tract or the lungs, it is believed that the soothing action of marshmallow on these areas is through a reflex action in the nervous system of the gut. In other words, the soothing demulcent action of the mucilage on the gut triggers a similar response in other mucous membranes throughout the body. Herbalist Matthew Wood (2004) notes that marshmallow root helps to calm the passages through which kidney and gallstones travel. In general, marshmallow's cooling and moistening energetics make it useful for soothing inflamed tissues and diminishing swelling (Easley & Horne, 2016).

Diarrhoea and constipation

Marshmallow root also helps the gut by providing a source of prebiotics to feed the beneficial bacteria that populate the gut. In addition, it is helpful for both diarrhoea and constipation, depending on how it is prepared. For diarrhoea, soak powdered root in just a small amount of cold water for at least an hour and then drink the mucilaginous result; the small amount of water used in this process will leave the rest of the powder capable of absorbing more water in the gut. For constipation, a teaspoon of powder can be soaked in 8 fluid ounces of cold water to form a fibre drink to help move gut contents out of the system.

Marshmallow may delay absorption of other drugs taken at the same time (Hoffmann, 2003).

Marshmallow recipes

Gut support tea

There is evidence that gastrointestinal inflammation and damage is linked to autoimmune conditions (Bone & Mills, 2013). This tea contains herbs that help to reduce inflammation and promote healing of the gastrointestinal tract and thus may be helpful for individuals suffering from a variety of autoimmune conditions. Both calendula (*Calendula officinalis*) flower and liquorice (*Glycyrrhiza glabra*) root are anti-inflammatory. Marshmallow (*Althaea officinalis*) root and liquorice are rich in mucilage that soothes tissue. Plantain (*Plantago* spp.) is also a demulcent herb, but its main action in this tea is as a mucous membrane trophorestorative that helps reduce gut permeability.

2g (0.07 oz) liquorice (*Glycyrrhiza glabra*) root

2g (0.07 oz) plantain (*Plantago* spp.) leaf

1g (0.04 oz) calendula (*Calendula officinalis*) flower

1g (0.04 oz) marshmallow (*Althaea officinalis*) root powder

1. Add liquorice, plantain and calendula to a heat-safe teapot, French press or glass jar.

2. Add 355 ml (12 fl oz) boiling water and leave to steep for an hour, or ideally overnight in a cool place.

3. Strain, stir in the marshmallow root powder, and let sit for an additional 15–30 minutes.

4. Stir again and drink.

Marshmallow vanilla lip balm

2 parts marshmallow (*Althaea officinalis*) root infused oil

2 parts shea butter

1 part vanilla bean (*Vanilla planifolia*) seed infused oil

½ part castor oil

1–2 parts beeswax (pastilles or grated)

A drop of Vitamin E oil (optional)

1. Measure oils and butter and place in a heat-safe bowl over a small saucepan of simmering water over low heat. Be careful not to splash any water into the mixture.

2. Weigh beeswax and add to the warmed oil and butter mixture. Continue to heat the mixture (over low heat), stirring with a sanitised, dry spoon until the beeswax has melted.

3. Pour into sanitised, dry tins or lip balm tubes and let cool.

4. Once cool, put the lids on and label the containers.

5. Store in a cool, dark place for up to 1 year.

Safety considerations

Marshmallow may delay absorption of other drugs taken at the same time (Hoffmann, 2003

MILK THISTLE

Silybum marianum

The Schools' Collection, Volume 0687, Page 0087

Local Cures collection from Miss Neill
Whillow: scum of buttermilk and fine oatmeal made into a paste and applied as poultice.
Whooping cough: Leaf of certain thistle boiled in new milk
Mumps: Walk the patient round the inside of a big pigsty three times
Worms: Tansy boiled in new new milk and given to the patient
Sty: Get 9 gooseberry thorns point 8 of them at the sty and throw away the 9th one you left shoulder
Blood:
(1) 3 feeds of boiled nettles in the early summer is supposed to be an excellent tonic. The leaves are boiled like cabbage. and prepared for consumption in the same way.
(2) Another home made blood purifier and made used in this district is ; cream of tartar sulphur treacle mixed into a syrup.

The whole family takes a spoonful of this mixture, It prevents boils, pimples and all skin blemishes.

The Schools' Collection, Volume 0572, Page 0298

Snarlús is an herb which grows on the ground and has a blossom of black nobs. Commonly called Soldiers. People boil it, put the juice into milk & give it to delicate children to drink.
Milk Thistle is a kind of soft thistle. If you squeeze the juice of it, it is like milk and when rubbed to warts will take them away.
The Buttercup does harm to land for tillage but if cows eat it, it will make the milk and butter good.
There is a weed which grows on piers or ruins of old houses. It has a small leaf and a pink blossom, & is supposed to cure Murrain in cows.
Camimile is a weed which grows in boggy places. To make a poultice of it & poppy heads, & apply to mumps or a sore ear as a sure remedy.

The Schools' Collection, Volume 1088, Page 0055

The milk thistle is good for warts, you squeeze the milk on the wart three times.

The Schools' Collection, Volume 0687, Page 0087

Whooping cough: Leaf of certain thistle boiled in new milk

The Schools' Collection, Volume 0572, Page 0298

Milk Thistle is a kind of soft thistle. If you squeeze the juice of it, it is like milk and when rubbed to warts will take them away.

The Schools' Collection, Volume 1088, Page 0055

The milk thistle is good for warts, you squeeze the milk on the wart three times.

Research showing that its constituents protect liver cells from chemical damage supports milk thistle's reputation as a liver tonic.

Safety considerations

Foster (2009) suggests dosing milk thistle for 4–8 weeks at a time, while other herbalists do not propose a maximum period of time. Individuals who have allergic reactions to plants in the thistle/daisy family (Asteraceae) may experience reactions to milk thistle. It is also possible that milk thistle may interfere with the use of insulin and other medications used for hypoglycemia (McIntyre, n.d.). No side effects or drug interactions have been reported (Hoffmann, 2003).

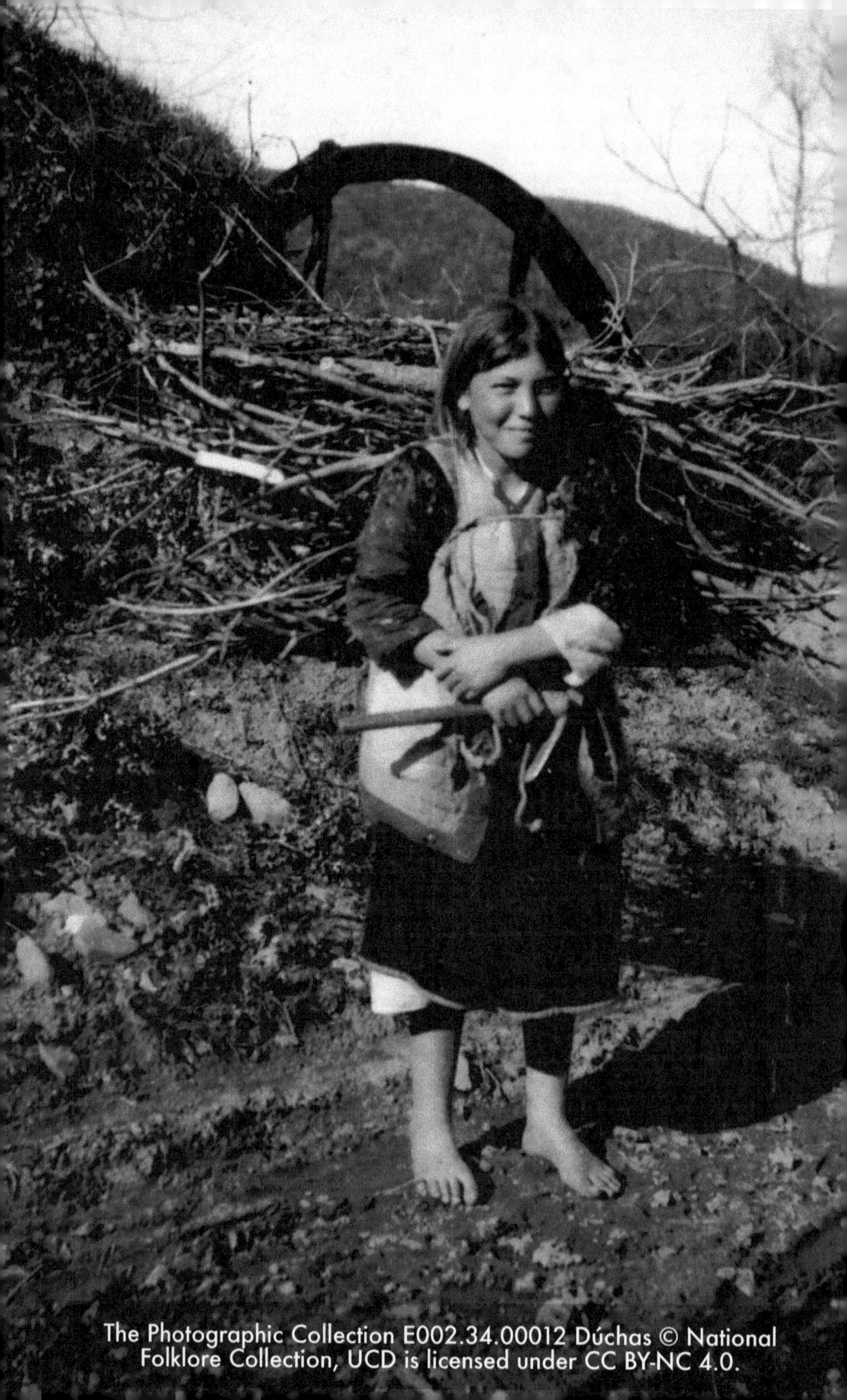

MUGWORT

Artemisia vulgaris

The Schools' Collection, Volume 0057, Page 0126

Mugwort is strong enough to intoxicate people. It is an old saying, If a footman put mugwort in his boots in the morning he may go 40 miles before noon and not be weary.
Bluebell bulbs will yield starch and was used for such in olden times it also makes a marvellous paste for books and is a known remedy for bald heads for producing hair or for beardless men.
Dandelion with Globe of down. The Schoolboys clock in everytown – It is also called Shepherds clock since the blossoms open and close at regular hours, and it tells when rain is near when the down flies of stem on a calm day.
Nettles boiled are a splendid tonic for the blood, and feed for pigs and ducks.
Fleabane laid on bites or stings cures them and keeps down the swelling

Stiffness and swelling - joint pain

The Schools' Collection, Volume 0057, Page 0128

Mugwort removes stiffness from joints also swelling of the feet and adds fragrance to a bath. It should be boiled and bathe joints in it.

In *An Irish Herbal,* Michael Scott writes,

> It [mugwort] grows along the borders of fields, in highways and waste places, and it flowers in June. If pounded and applied with the oil of sweet almonds, it cures the pain of the stomach. If the juice is mixed with oil of roses and applied, it will ease pains or aches in the joints and cramps. It also provokes menstruation. If it is added to barrels of ale, it will prevent them from souring (Scott, 1986).

Mugwort – other uses

Mugwort can be used as a bitter to stimulate the digestive system. The herb's volatile oils provide carminative effects in addition to stimulating the sense of bitterness, which aids in digestion. Its mild nervine activity, which also appears to be related to its volatile oil concentration, may help ease depression and stress. Additionally, mugwort can be used as an emmenagogue to encourage normal menstrual flow (Hoffmann, 2003).

Mugwort recipes

Mugwort, chicory and tangerine digestive bitters

Can be taken by the dropperful before meals.

1 tbsp (½ fl oz) raw honey

1 cup (8 fl oz) chicory (*Cichorium intybus*) root tincture

¼ cup (2 fl oz) lemon balm (*Melissa officinalis*) tincture

⅛ cup (1 fl oz) mugwort (*Artemisia vulgaris*) tincture

1 fresh tangerine, chopped (peel included)

1. Blend honey and tinctures together in a clean, pint-sized glass canning jar.
2. Add the chopped tangerine.
3. Place a square piece of natural waxed paper on top of the jar, then seal the jar with a lid.
4. Cap tightly and give a shake to ensure that ingredients are thoroughly mixed.
5. Let macerate for 1 week.
6. Line a wire strainer with a few layers of cheesecloth, or simply place the cheesecloth within a clean funnel placed in the mouth of a jar, and decant the mixture.
7. Strain the mixture through the cheesecloth and with clean, dry hands, gather the cloth up and squeeze strongly, squeezing as much liquid from the marc as possible.
8. Transfer the liquid into clean, dark-coloured glass bottles using a clean funnel.
9. Label and store in a cool, dark place for up to 1 year.
10. Take 1 dropperful 3x/day (before meals) or add to mixed drinks.

Beard oil

With antimicrobial, skin-soothing properties.

3 parts mugwort (*Artemisia vulgaris*) leaf infused oil

½ part sage (*Salvia officinalis*) leaf infused oil

3 drops eucalyptus (*Eucalyptus globulus*) essential oil

1. See "How to make a herbal infused oil" (page 46).
2. Add the herbal oils and eucalyptus essential oil to a dark-coloured, sanitised, dry glass container.
3. Cover and shake well to combine.
4. Label, and store in a cool, dark place for up to 1 year.
5. To use, apply 5–7 drops to your hands, rub through your beard, and add more as needed.

Safety considerations

Mugwort is potentially allergenic to people sensitive to plants in the Asteraceae family (Hoffmann, 2003).

MULLEIN

Verbascum thapsus

The Schools' Collection, Volume 0219, Page 0111

A great many herbs grow in Barnacoola, and nearly every one of them are of some use. The following is a list of some of the herbs which are found growing in this parish:- Dandelion, watercress, cumphery, clover, balm, docking root, marshmallow, garlic, ivy leaves, purple daisies and the jaundice herb.

The dandelion herb is good for a bad stomach. It is also used for making wines.

Docks cure the sting of an nettle by rubbing the juice of the dock on the place where the sting is.

Plantain leaf cures a sore, by putting the leaf to the sore and putting the bandage outside of it.

To boil the root of the mullen plant and make a plaster of it is good to heal any kind of a sore.

Nettles contain a large amount of iron and when boiled like cabbage are very good for the health.

> **Dandelion leaves boiled and the water strained into some vesell and to drink the water is good for anyone who has diseased liver and the leaves when boiled are given**
>
> The Schools' Collection, Volume 0219, Page 0111
>
> **To boil the root of the mullen plant and make a plaster of it is good to heal any kind of a sore.**

Used since ancient times, mullein was described by Culpeper to address everything from cramps and coughs to rough (but not smooth) warts and gout (Culpeper, 1653).

An oil for earaches is made from the stalk and blossoms. Mullein leaves have been utilised in cough remedies for bronchial and respiratory infections, asthma and glandular imbalances. The leaves are used as an infusion or as a tincture.

Mullein is a helpful respiratory treatment. The plant promotes fluid production and decreases inflammation, which makes expectoration easier. It is believed to be helpful for bronchitis, which is characterised by a painful and harsh cough. It is used to treat tracheal inflammation and associated conditions because of its anti-inflammatory and demulcent qualities. An extract prepared by infusing mullein flowers in olive oil is noted for external use to relieve ear issues.

Mullein recipes

Mullein flower oil

Warmed and added into the ear with a clean spoon twice daily, this works for earaches. See "Earache oil recipe", page 114.

Breathe easy decongestion chest oil

2 parts mullein (*Verbascum thapsus*) leaf and / or flower infused oil

1 part yarrow (*Achillea millefolium*) aerial parts infused oil

3 drops of eucalyptus (*Eucalyptus globulus*) essential oil

1. See "How to make a herbal infused oil" (page 46).
2. Measure the appropriate amount of each herbal oil and transfer to a dark-coloured. sanitised, dry glass container.
3. Cover and shake well to combine.
4. Label, and store in a cool, dark place for up to 1 year.
5. To use, massage a small amount over chest and upper back as needed.

Safety considerations

No side effects or drug interactions have been reported.

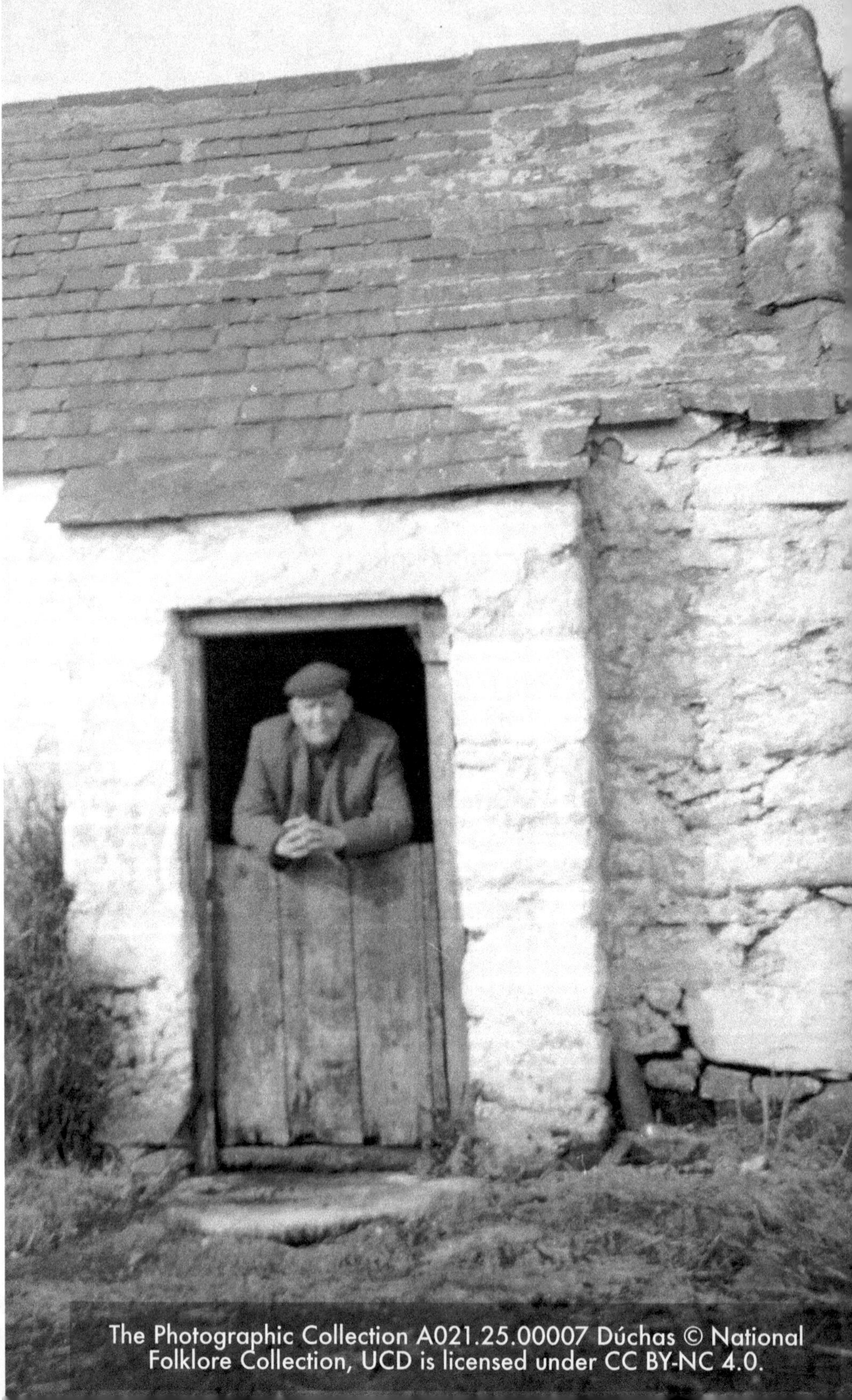

NETTLE

Urtica dioica

The Schools' Collection, Volume 0022, Page 0402

The nettles are good for rheumatism. The way the nettles are used to cure rheumatism is to boil them and drink the juice.

The Schools' Collection, Volume 0027, Page 0097

Herbs are roots found in bad land some are dangerous and some more very good. Most herbs are dangerous to sheep but the goat eats any kind. The farmers long ago used to put goats in amongst sheep so that they would eat the dangerous herbs. Long ago the doctors used to mix and boil herbs and make medicines. Nettles boiled and dandelions boiled were one of their many cures for ringworm. They were supposed to have charms.

The Schools' Collection, Volume 0049, Page 0171

Nettles are boiled for pigs and fowl. They are also boiled for people who have a rash on them. There is castor oil in daisies.

Where ever a nettle grows there is always a dock leaf growing beside it. Dock leaves are used for the curing of stings from a nettle.

The Schools' Collection, Volume 0050, Page 0401

Nettles are used for curing warts and is also good for ducklings.

The Schools' Collection, Volume 0050, Page 0470

Nettle Seed – Useful in chest infections and as a blood medicine.

The Schools' Collection, Volume 0051, Page 0163

Nettle:- It was believed that if people ate three meals of nettles in the month of March that they would have no sickness during the year.

The Schools' Collection, Volume 0056, Page 0151

Nettles were used as a cure for Rheumatism by placing them between two sheets.

The Schools' Collection, Volume 0057, Pages 0122-0123

The common stinging nettle is a well known cure for rash. The seeds or little knots can be boiled and the water used in cases of constipation. It is also a cure for bladder disease.

When stung with a nettle the country people all know that they should rub the affected part with dock leaf and strange both it is remarked grow side by side. Dock is a very useful herb and it is so called from the colour of its roots which is the most valuable part of the plant. It is used for hemorrhage of the lungs. The best way of using it as a remedy is, wash roots and boil half a pound of the powdered root in a pint of golden syrup. This can then be taken in teaspoonful doses. It is also used in liver complaints and is a mild laxative.

Nettles boiled are a splendid tonic for the blood, and feed for pigs and ducks.

The Schools' Collection, Volume 0077, Page 064

There are not as many cures now as there were long ago.
My Grandmother told me a few.
(1) Nettles are very good to eat during the month of March, and it is said that you should boil them and eat them three times during the month, and the person that does this will not get any disease during the year.
(2) The roots of docket leaves boiled in milk are used to cure a sick stomach.
(3) Garlic boiled in milk is good for a cold, and to put some into your shoes would cure rheumatism.

The Schools' Collection, Volume 0079, Page 0296

Nettles are a great blood purifier, also dandelion. Dandelion tea cures bronchitis and other diseases. Meacan na gcaorach cures mumps, and a very good cough cure can also be made by boiling the roots.
Young nettles and dandelion leaves are cooked and eaten like cabbage greens. Boglas cures boils and all kinds of open sores. It is mixed with oatmeal and used as a poultice. Garlick boiled and mixed with bad whiskey is a great cure for a cough.

Rheumatism

The Schools' Collection, Volume 0022, Page 0402

The way the nettles are used to cure rheumatism is to boil them and drink the juice.

The Schools' Collection, Volume 0056, Page 0151

Nettles were used as a cure for Rheumatism by placing them between two sheets.

Nettle stimulates the kidneys to increase excretion of uric acid, which aids in easing arthritis and gout (McIntyre, 1996). Nettle has a long history as support for these imbalances. As noted in *The Lancet* (Volume 355, 3 June 2000):

> A clinical trial in which osteoarthritis patients topically applied a nettle extract cream to painful joints concluded that stinging nettle could prove beneficial for pain relief and modification of the disease process (Rayburn et al., 2009). After a week, patients with osteoarthritic pain at the base of their thumb or index finger who received stinging nettle leaf applied to the area reported pain and disability reductions that were noticeably higher than those who received a placebo, according to another clinical study (Randall et al., 2000).

Ringworm

The Schools' Collection, Volume 0027, Page 0097

Long ago the doctors used to mix and boil herbs and make medicines. Nettles boiled and dandelions boiled were one of their many cures for ringworm.

Rash

The Schools' Collection, Volume 0049, Page 0171

Nettles are boiled for pigs and fowl. They are also boiled for people who have a rash on them.

The Schools' Collection, Volume 0057, Page 0122

The common stinging nettle is a well-known cure for rash. The seeds or little knots can be boiled and the water used in cases of consumption. It is also a cure for bladder disease.

As an alterative, nettle cleanses the blood and helps the body absorb nutrients and proteins, neutralise acid and get rid of waste.

As such, it can be used to balance blood toxicity, arthritis, gout, rheumatism, eczema and skin problems resulting from metabolic disorders by detoxifying the body of metabolic wastes (Holmes, 1997).

Warts

The Schools' Collection, Volume 0050, Page 0401

Nettles are used for curing warts and is also good for ducklings.

Formic acid is an antiseptic, biodegradable organic acid that is colourless but has a strong, irritating smell. The acid is corrosive but is mainly used in wart treatments because it dries out the warts from the wart roots. In nature, formic acid can be found in very high concentrations in stinging nettles.

Chest infections and blood

The Schools' Collection, Volume 0050, Page 0470

Nettle Seed - Useful in chest infections and as a blood medicine.

The Schools' Collection, Volume 0079, Page 0296

Nettles are a great blood purifier, also dandelion. Dandelion tea cures bronchitis and other diseases.

This illustrates nettle's reputation as a healthful herbal tonic that is suitable for everyday consumption. Nettle energises and supports the entire body. Nettle also provides the body with nourishment, especially for the blood. "Chlorophyll and red blood cells have nearly identical molecular structures; the only difference is that chlorophyll contains magnesium where haemoglobin contains iron," notes herbalist Robin Rose Bennett (2014).

Tonic

The Schools' Collection, Volume 0051, Page 0163

> Nettle: It was believed that if people ate three meals of nettles in the month of March that they would have no sickness during the year.

The Schools' Collection, Volume 0057, Page 0126

> Nettles boiled are a splendid tonic for the blood, and feed for pigs and ducks.

The Schools' Collection, Volume 0077, Page 0064

> There are not as many cures now as there were long ago. My Grandmother told me a few.
> (1) Nettles are very good to eat during the month of March, and it is said that you should boil them and eat them three times during the month, and the person that does this will not get any disease during the year.

This embodies all that is well-known and cherished about nettle, such as its ability to balance anaemia, promote recovery from illness, and build blood.

Nettle is a super-nourisher, high in vitamins and minerals, especially iron and calcium. In addition to nourishment, nettle is also an alterative that helps to detoxify the body and is used as a spring tonic. Examples of how to incorporate nettle into the diet include drinking it as a nourishing infusion, steaming or sautéing the tops of spring nettles and using them as you would any green leafy vegetable, or juicing the leaves and stalks to make a green juice.

Nettle is also an excellent remedy for allergies and hay fever. Nettle is useful for 'growing pains' in young children, when their bones and joints ache. Nettle is excellent as a reproductive tonic for men and women and can be used as a hair and scalp tonic (Gladstar, 2012).

The rich nutrition of nettle soothes fatigue. Another advantage of nettle is that it can help keep blood sugar levels stable; studies show that nettle contains both hypoglycaemic and hyperglycaemic ingredients (Hoffmann, 2003). Nettle leaf extract was shown to enhance glycaemic control in type-2 diabetic patients requiring insulin therapy in a clinical trial (Kianbakht et al., 2013).

Nettle is a deeply nourishing tonic for the adrenals and kidneys. Nettle seed has been used as a restorative tonic for the kidneys (Winston & Maimes, 2019), while some consume the seed to strengthen the adrenal glands and provide energy during times of fatigue (Kress, 2004). Finnish herbalist Henriette Kress (2004) suggests consuming 1–2 tablespoons of nettle seed per day in yogurt or thick juice.

Nettle can be useful in cases of hay fever, asthma and seasonal allergies through its anti-inflammatory and antihistamine actions (Easley & Horne, 2016). Nettle has been used for addressing allergies and other respiratory issues such as coughs, asthma and bronchitis (Garrett, 2003). Mittman (1990) conducted a clinical study in which more than half of patients suffering from allergic rhinitis reported symptom abatement after taking a freeze-dried stinging nettle leaf preparation, while all treated patients reported symptom improvement. Helms & Miller (2006) suggest that nettle's anti-inflammatory action may be attributable to its histamine content, and suggest an adult dose of 300 mg twice daily of freeze-dried nettle leaf.

In terms of animal health, nettles were used for fluke in cattle and added to meal for fowl, especially turkeys and ducks.

Bladder

The Schools' Collection, Volume 0057, Page 0122

It is also a cure for bladder disease.

Nettle leaf and root may assist with issues involving the kidneys and genitourinary system. Both are diuretic, helping to flush the urinary system and remove toxins. Nettle eases urinary discomfort and is tonic and strengthening to the kidneys, improving overall vitality. The herb is used to soften and expel kidney stones and gravel from the urinary tract, as well as to soothe fluid retention, cystitis, urethritis and prostatitis. Nettle root is used to decongest the prostate in the case of benign prostatic hyperplasia (BPH) (Holmes, 1997) and reduce urinary tract symptoms caused by an enlarged prostate gland pressing on the urethra. A decoction made with only the stem of the nettle plant has been used to address difficult urination related to prostate issues (Young et al., 2015).

In a clinical trial designed to study root extract of *Urtica dioica* for lower urinary tract symptoms resulting from BPH, 81% of patients who received the nettle extract reported improved symptoms compared with 16% in the placebo group, and the nettle group also experienced a modest decrease in prostate size (Safarinejad, 2005). Foster (1993) reports that several clinical studies found that nettle extract reduced the frequency of need to pass urine in the night in patients with less severe prostate enlargement. Hoffmann (2003) cites studies that showed improved urine flow as well as reduced urinary frequency and volume after taking nettle root.

Measles

The Schools' Collection, Volume 0079, Page 0354

Nettles, is a cure for measles.

Historically, nettle tea was deemed to cure measles. In this instance, the nettles are boiled with very little water, strained and sugar or salt added to the liquid. It is then drunk by the patient. Another method was to boil the nettles in whiskey after which it was strained, and the liquid given to the sufferer.

Nettle is a pleasant-tasting food and is often steamed and served as a mineral-rich addition to meals. It can be used to replace spinach in any recipe, but must always be well steamed as it will sting if undercooked. It can be served as a tea to prevent allergic attacks (Gladstar, 2012).
Fresh nettles were often eaten in the same way as cabbage. They were also mixed with mashed potatoes to make a nettle champ or colcannon.

A bottle of nettle juice would be kept in the house as a regular traditional medicine, and boiled leaves were sometimes taken in milk. These remedies were used for blood pressure, stomach trouble, pimples, bad breath, varicose veins and dull eyes. The nettle leaves were also applied to rashes, sores or abscesses.

Boiled nettle roots were thought to help pleurisy. As well as being reputed to be particularly effective against measles, nettles were also called into direct use for whooping cough.

Nettle recipes

Nettle soup (serves 6)

45g butter

285g potatoes, peeled and chopped

110g onions, chopped

110g leeks, chopped

1 litre homemade chicken or vegetable stock

140g young nettles (*Urtica dioica*), washed and chopped

150ml full-fat milk

Sea salt and freshly ground black pepper

1. Melt the butter in a heavy-bottomed saucepan, and when it foams, add the potatoes, onions and leeks, tossing them in the butter until well coated.

2. Sprinkle with salt and freshly ground pepper.

3. Cover with the saucepan lid. Sweat over a gentle heat for 10 minutes or until the vegetables are soft.

4. Add the stock and boil until the vegetables are just cooked, then add the nettle leaves.

5. Simmer uncovered for just a few minutes.

6. Try not to overcook the vegetables or they will lose their flavour.

7. Add the milk and liquidise.

8. Season to taste.

9. Serve hot with a drizzle of nettle pesto, if available.

Nettle shampoo

180–240 ml (6–8 fl oz) herbal infusion of nettle (*Urtica dioica*) leaf

90 ml (3 fl oz) liquid castile soap

1.5 ml (0.05 fl oz) carrier oil of choice such as jojoba oil or sweet almond oil (more can be added for dry hair or less for oily hair)

30–40 drops essential oil of choice

1. Make herbal infusion, using 7–15 g (0.25–0.5 oz) of herb per 240 ml (8 fl oz) water.

2. Let steep for 4 hours, then strain.

3. Combine essential oil and carrier oil in a jar or squeeze bottle and mix well.

4. Add strained infusion and castile soap, cap, and shake.

5. Shake bottle before using.

6. If shampoo is not going to be used within a few weeks, refrigerate.

Nourishing hair oil

1 part nettle (*Urtica dioica*) leaf infused oil

1 part rosemary (*Salvia rosmarinus*) leaf infused oil

1. See "How to make a herbal infused oil" (page 46).
2. Add the herbal oils to a dark-coloured, sanitised, dry glass container.
3. Cover and shake well to combine.
4. Label, and store in a cool, dark place for up to 1 year.
5. Use a dropper to apply about 1–2 tsp of oil directly to the scalp. Massage gently for a few minutes, then leave on for at least 30 minutes or overnight before washing. Use 1–3 times per week for best results.

Digestive, liver and allergy tea

1 tbsp burdock (*Arctium lappa*) root

1 tbsp dandelion (*Taraxacum officinale*) root

1 tbsp nettle (*Urtica dioica*) leaf

1 tbsp red clover (*Trifolium pratense*) flowers

1 quart water

1. Place nettle, dandelion leaf and red clover in a tea pot or flask, and set aside.
2. In a a quart of water in a covered saucepan, bring the burdock and dandelion root to a boil. Immediately lower the heat, and simmer for 20 minutes.

3. Pour the hot root decoction over the nettle, dandelion leaf and red clover.

4. Steep for at least 20 minutes and up to 4 hours before straining.

5. Drink throughout the day and store any remaining tonic in the fridge for up to 24 hours.

Nettle vinegar

Dried nettle (*Urtica dioica*) leaf

Raw, unpasteurised, organic apple cider vinegar

1. Fill a clean, dry glass jar ¼ full of dried nettle leaf.

2. Pour enough apple cider vinegar to fill the jar, ensuring nettle leaf is covered by a couple of inches.

3. Cover the jar with a small piece of parchment paper to prevent the vinegar coming into contact with any metal, and cap with a lid.

4. Let this mixture sit in a cool, dark location for 3–6 weeks. Shake occasionally and add extra vinegar as needed to prevent the herb from poking out above the liquid.

5. Strain and reserve.

6. If stored properly in a cool, dark cabinet, your nettle vinegar should last a year.

Basic vinaigrette dressing

3 parts cold-pressed extra virgin olive oil or oil of your choice

1 part nettle vinegar

Fresh herbs of your choice, minced (2–4 tbsp per cup of dressing)

Salt and pepper to taste

1. Combine all ingredients in a clean, glass jar.
2. Shake well, label, and store in the fridge.

Safety considerations

Fresh nettle causes urticaria if applied topically. Internal use may theoretically decrease the efficacy of anticoagulant drugs (Hoffmann, 2003).

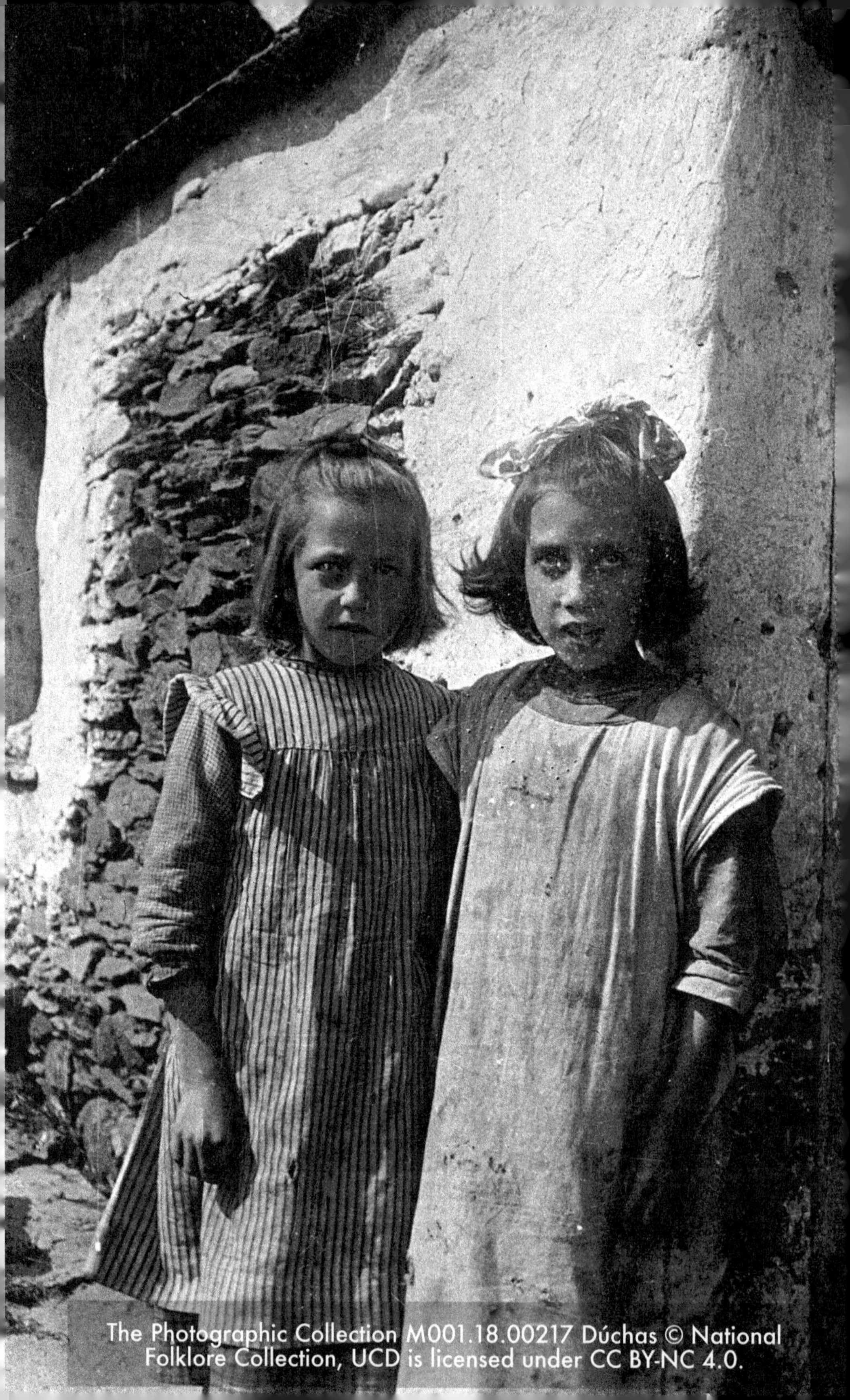

PARSLEY

Petroselinum crispum

The Schools' Collection, Volume 0690, Page 0114

"Burst Leaf" boiled in lard and applied to a burst or bruise will give immediate relief.
Rat Tail leaf: a poultice applied for a headache. Soothing and cooling.
Marsh Mallow leaf boiled will cure a sprain.
Parsley leaf is the cure of kidney and liver disease.
Ivy leaf.
Boiled ivy leaves will cure chilblains. Get nine ivy leaves and rub them to warts saying "In the name of the father Son and Holy Ghost" then place them where no one will walk and when they will decay the warts will disappearing.
Ivy leaves applied to a cut corn will prevent it from festering.

The Schools' Collection, Volume 0121, Page 0028

Long ago, many were the old cures practised by the people.

> The juice of the dandelion was said to be a cure for any disease of the liver. Parsley and gin mixed is a cure for kidney trouble. The juice of red ivy is said to be a cure for corns. Common earth mixed with water is a cure for a sting of a bee or wasp. The juice of house-leek is said to be a cure for sore eyes.
>
> The Schools' Collection, Volume 0690, Page 0114

> Parsley leaf is the cure of kidney and liver disease.
>
> The Schools' Collection, Volume 0121, Page 0028

> Parsley and gin mixed is a cure for kidney trouble.

One of parsley's primary historical herbal indications is for bladder and kidney health, especially when it comes to stones. Parsley's long-standing reputation for breaking up deposits in the bladder or kidneys appears to go back as far as Roman antiquity: Pliny the Elder (77/1906) remarked that the seed of *Apium* was a diuretic and that the seed or root in wine broke bladder stones. *Apium* was applied topically with egg white or boiled in water and drunk for kidney issues (Pliny, 77/1906). The root and seed of a type of parsley called *oreoselinon,* taken as a libation in wine, were also used as a diuretic (Dioscorides, 70/2000).

Cherokee tribes have used parsley in infusion of leaves and roots for kidneys, dropsy and bladder issues (Hamel & Chiltoskey, 1975; Native American Ethnobotany Database, 2003) and European settlers of Appalachia also employed it as a diuretic for kidney inflammation (Garrett, 2003). The Mi'kmaq have traditionally used parsley as a urinary aid in instances of cold being present in the bladder (Chandler et al., 1979; Native American Ethnobotany Database, 2003).

Parsley is very rich in calcium, iron and various trace elements. Taken in any form it is beneficial to the kidneys and the urinary tract. It also stimulates blood circulation. A decoction of the dried root is particularly good for sluggishness of the kidney and, as a result, combats gravel, urine retention and arthritis, as well as dropsy and jaundice. Parsley tea was used successfully during the First World War to treat men in the trenches who had developed kidney complications from dysentery. An infusion of the fresh leaves has a regulatory effect on menstrual discharge and in the process helps to relieve associated pains and cramps (Harford, 2019).

Parsley recipes

Wild mushroom cream sauce (serves 8)

50g (2oz) butter

175g (6oz) onion, finely chopped

450g (1lb) wild mushrooms (chanterelles, morels, ceps, false chanterelles or the common field mushroom), sliced

Salt and freshly ground pepper

Squeeze of lemon juice

225ml (8fl oz) cream

Freshly chopped parsley (*Petroselinum crispum*)

1 tbsp freshly chopped chives (optional)

1. Melt half the butter in a heavy saucepan until the butter foams.
2. Add the chopped onion in a bowl, cover and sweat over low heat for 5 to 10 minutes, or until it is soft but not coloured.
3. In the meantime, if needed, sauté the sliced mushrooms in batches in a heated frying pan with the remaining butter.
4. Add salt, freshly ground pepper and a small squeeze of lemon juice to each batch.

5. Add the mushrooms to the onions in the saucepan, then add the cream and allow to bubble for a few minutes.

6. Taste and correct the seasoning, and add the chopped herbs.

Safety considerations

Not for use in pregnancy. Be very careful foraging cow parsley owing to its close resemblance to deadly hemlock.

RIBWORT PLANTAIN

Plantago lanceolata

The Schools' Collection, Volume 0051, Page 0163

The most harmful weeds in this district are groundsel, crows' foot, nightshade, dandelion robin run the hedge and the thistle - the three last named grow in good land.

Many herbs are used for medicinal purposes The green leaves of the dandelion were eaten for liver complaint. Children collected the leaves which were pounded in a pestle-mortar - a little whiskey was added to the bruised leaves and the mixture was put into a bottle and given to the children to drink.

Nettle: It was believed that if people ate three meals of nettles in the month of March that they would have no sickness during the year.

Ribgrass was used in making a green ointment for healing burns. Ribgrass, chopped laurel leaves, yarrow & lard were boiled together for 2 or 3 hours & the green ointment was the result.

The purging plant was a green shrub - cattle were fond of it.

Another herb called the meacan buidhe (I do not know it) was scraped & boiled in milk.
If scraped on both sides it was deadly [posionous]

Burns

The Schools' Collection, Volume 0051, Page 0163

Ribgrass was used in making a green ointment for healing burns. Ribgrass, chopped laurel leaves, yarrow & lard were boiled together for 2 or 3 hours & the green ointment was the result.

This recipe is hardly surprising given that plantain is one of Western herbalism's primary topical healing agents, used as a lotion, ointment, compress or poultice for cuts and bruises. It may be applied topically for haemorrhoids and skin ulcerations.

Plantain is an effective herb for bites, stings, cuts and scrapes, and it helps to draw out slivers, splinters or stingers (Bruton-Seal & Seal, 2008). Plantain may also be used to soothe and cool the pain, itching, or burning symptoms of poison ivy, nettles or sunburn.

Plantain's anti-inflammatory and astringent properties are applicable to soothe and tone other chronic or acute skin conditions such as eczema, rosacea, shingles, varicose veins and haemorrhoids (Bruton-Seal & Seal, 2008). The root is sometimes used like comfrey for its bone-knitting properties (Blair, 2014).

Plantain – other uses

Plantain may be beneficial for coughs and mild bronchitis because it soothes irritated and sore membranes and functions as a mild expectorant. Its astringent properties aid with haemorrhoids, diarrhoea and bleeding cystitis.

Plantain has been used for the internal treatment of diseases of the blood including syphilis, specific or non-specific glandular disease and mercurial poisoning (Ellingwood, 1919).

Ribwort plantain or ribgrass grows in fields and meadows in May and June. It has a binding nature and has similar qualities to common plantain (*Plantago major*). It is particularly good for worms in children. The juice of it is given before the fit of an ague to prevent its approaching (Scott, 1986). Some herbalists suggest that plantain can be used as an emergency water purifier owing to its inhibition of *E. coli*, *Streptococcus pneumoniae* and *Giardia intestinalis* (giardia), as well as its anthelmintic properties and soothing effect on the digestive tract (Blair, 2014). Plantain may also be used in cases of candida overgrowth such as thrush (Grieve, 1931/1971).

Plantain has high nutritional value and is sometimes called the Green Bandage; it is among the best herbs for poultices.

Plantain seeds are frequently employed in laxative blends because of their soothing bulk action and high mucilage content. The psyllium seeds used in many laxatives are produced from a cultivated plantain (*Plantago afra*). Plantain may prove helpful for liver sluggishness and digestion inflammation (Gladstar, 2012).

Plantain recipes

Poultices and compresses

Poultices and compresses are a way of applying fresh plant material or a herbal infusion or decoction directly to the skin. Both preparations can accelerate the healing of wounds, bruises, bites and stings, burns, and soft tissue injury; calm skin conditions such as acne and eczema; promote circulation; and ease pain and inflammation.

Poultices are, simply, an application of plant material to the skin. Plants that are anti-inflammatory, vulnerary and/or astringent, and are easily found in abundance, such as self heal (*Prunella vulgaris*) aerial parts and violet (*Viola* spp.) aerial parts, are all good candidates for use in poultices. While poultices are most commonly made with fresh plant material (and this is the preferred method, when available), dried herbal powder can be mixed with water and applied directly to the skin as a paste. In addition to the actions mentioned above, poultices also excel at pulling material (e.g., splinters) and infection out of the skin – plantain leaf is a great candidate for this. Compresses are made by soaking a piece of cloth in a pre-made herbal preparation, such as an infusion. The soaked cloth is then applied to the affected area. Compresses are often preferred when fresh plant material is not available, and can be made with any infusion or decoction. Compresses can also be made with tincture, but because so much liquid is needed to bathe the cloth, this may not be a cost-effective option. Compresses are most commonly applied hot (this adds the benefit of stimulating circulation), but can also be useful cool, especially for burns, headaches and inflammation.

Materials needed

Fresh herbs or a herbal infusion or decoction

Clean cotton cloth

Knife and cutting board, blender / food processor, or mortar and pestle (optional)

Directions – poultice

1. Harvest fresh plant material and remove any debris.
2. Grind, chop or use the mortar and pestle to mash up the plant material with a bit of water.
3. Apply mashed-up plant material to the affected area.
4. Wrap clean cotton cloth around plant material to keep it in place.
5. Leave in place for several hours or as long as is comfortable, up to 12 hours.

Directions – compress

1. In a hot infusion or decoction, soak a clean cotton cloth.

2. Once cloth is still warm, but not too hot to touch, remove from liquid and gently squeeze, draining it of excess infusion/decoction, but keeping it as moist as possible.

3. Lay cloth on the affected area and either wrap with a dry cotton cloth or keep exposed.

4. Once the cloth cools, repeat as often as desired.

Bug bite and rash salve

4 parts plantain (*Plantago* spp.) leaf infused oil

4 parts lavender (*Lavandula* spp.) flower bud infused oil

1 part beeswax (pastilles or grated)

1. See "How to make a herbal infused oil" (page 46).

2. Measure the oils and place in a heat-safe bowl over a small saucepan of simmering water on a low heat. Be careful not to splash any water into the oil.

3. Weigh beeswax and add to the warmed oil. Continue to heat the mixture (over low heat), stirring with a sanitised, dry spoon until the beeswax has melted.

4. While warm, pour individual portions into sanitised salve tubes and allow to cool, uncapped, at room temperature.

5. Once cool, put the lids on and label the containers.

6. In a cool, dark place store for up to 1 year.

7. To use, apply to itchy areas of the skin and repeat as needed.

Soothing cuticle oil

1 part calendula (*Calendula officinalis*) flower infused oil

1 part lavender (*Lavandula* spp.) flower bud infused oil

1 part plantain (*Plantago* spp.) leaf infused oil

Vitamin E oil (optional, added at 0.5–1% dilution)

1. See "How to make a herbal infused oil" (page 46).
2. Add the herbal oils to a dark-coloured, sanitised, dry glass container.
3. Add vitamin E oil if using.
4. Cover and shake well to combine.
5. Label, store in a cool, dark place for up to 1 year.
6. To use, gently massage 1–2 drops into each cuticle.

Soothing lip balm

1 part calendula (*Calendula officinalis*) flower infused oil

2 parts shea butter

1 part plantain (*Plantago* spp.) leaf infused oil

½ part castor oil

1–2 parts beeswax (pastilles or grated)

Vitamin E oil (optional, added at 0.5%–1% dilution by volume)

1. Measure oils and butter and place in a heat-safe bowl or glass canning jar over a small saucepan of simmering water on a low heat. Be careful not to splash any water into the oil.

2. Weigh beeswax and add to the warmed oil. Continue to heat the mixture (over low heat), stirring with a sanitised, dry spoon until the beeswax has melted.

3. Remove from heat.

4. Pour into sanitised, dry tins or lip balm tubes and let cool.

5. Once cool, put the lids on and label the containers.

6. Store in a cool, dark place for up to 1 year.

Safety considerations

No side effects or drug interactions have been reported (Hoffmann, 2003).

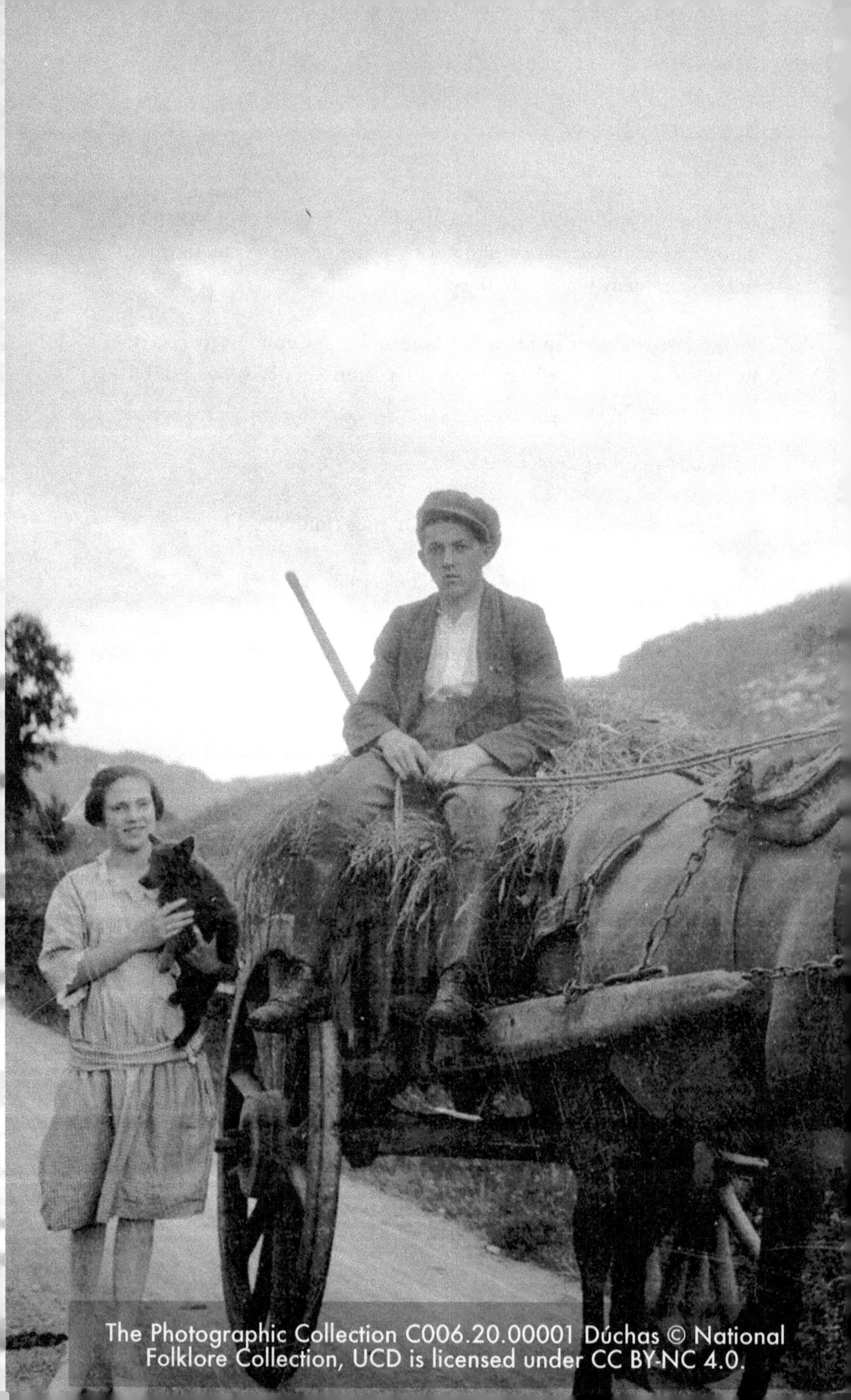

SORREL

Rumex acetosa

The Schools' Collection, Volume 0687, Page 0147

Cures collected from Mrs Reilly Johnstown aged 75.
Wood sorrel chopped up finely mixed with lard is good for sores of every description
For Boils: Plantain leaf for boils and swellings. Take out the tough veins of the leaf and chop finely. Make some oatmeal gruel and pour over the chopped leaves. Apply as an ointment. The whole leaf is also applied to cuts.
The Lady's mantle: A plant which used to grow in the vicinity was an infallible cure for burns. It was chopped and mixed with unsalted butter. The Blessed Virgin is supposed to have touched it sometime hence its virtue.
Leaves of the elder tree boiled in oatmeal and water was good for boils and swellings of any kind.

The Schools' Collection, Volume 0687, Page 0147

Wood sorrel chopped up finely mixed with lard is good for sores of every description.

Common sorrel was believed to be a "cooling" herb and helpful for swellings and inflammatory conditions. It has been used to treat jaundice, internal ulcers, fevers and skin tumours. Common sorrel also had a number of common uses such as treating wounds, sores, bruises, boils and chickenpox.

Sorrel recipes

Forager's soup

50g (2oz) butter

110g (4oz) onion, diced

150g (5oz) potatoes, diced

600ml (1 pint) chicken stock, vegetable stock or hot water

425–600ml (¾–1 pint) creamy milk (use ¼ cream and ¾ milk), brought to boiling point

250g (9oz) chopped wild greens (nettles, wild sorrel, young dandelions, wild garlic, borage, wild rocket, nasturtium leaves, poppy leaves, watercress)

Extra virgin olive oil

1. Melt the butter in a heavy-bottomed saucepan.
2. When the butter foams, add the diced onion and potatoes and toss until well coated.
3. Sprinkle with salt and freshly ground pepper.

4. Cover with a butter wrapper or piece of greaseproof paper (to trap the steam) and the saucepan lid, and sweat over a gentle heat for 10 minutes until the vegetables are almost soft but not coloured.

5. Discard the greaseproof paper and add the boiling milk and hot stock.

6. Return to the boil and continue cooking until the onions and potatoes are tender.

7. After adding the greens, boil them uncovered for two to three minutes, or until they are just cooked.

8. Do not overcook or the soup will lose its vibrant green colour.

9. Purée the soup in a liquidiser.

10. Taste and correct seasoning. serve, scattered with a few wild garlic flowers if available.

Safety considerations

Common sorrel is thought to contain oxalate crystals and is best not consumed in large quantities. Like other docks, sorrel can trigger hay fever or aggravate asthma in some people (Harford, 2019).

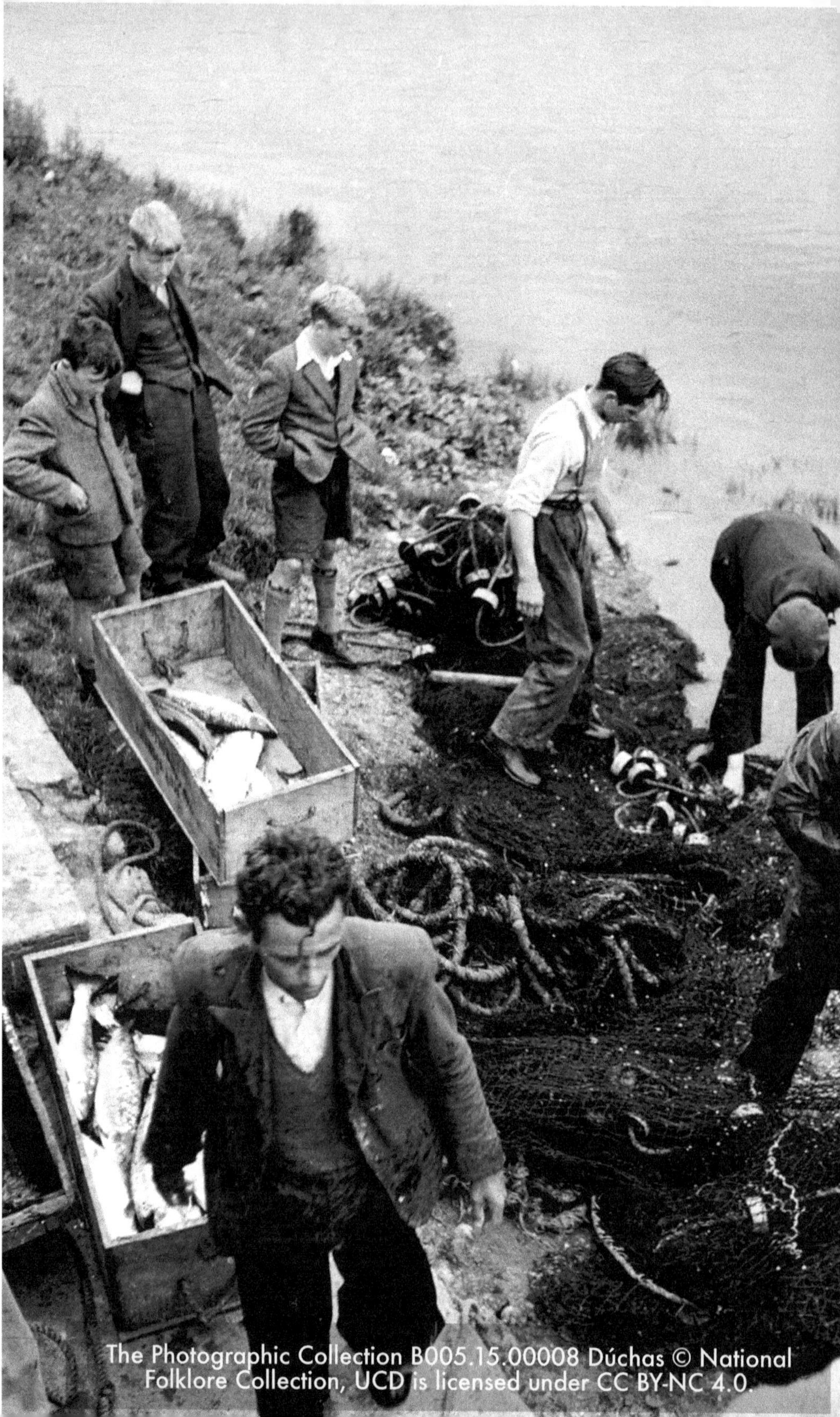

ST JOHN'S WORT

Hypericum perforatum.

The Schools' Collection, Volume 0029, Pages 0358-0359

In mostly every district in Ireland, herbs are to be found in abundance.

A week called 'chicken weed' causes much harm to the potato crop. It grows in the drills, and robs the potato of the food it needs.

The dandelion is reckoned to be a good cure for Rheumatism. It is boiled, and the juice is rubbed to the places where the Rheumatism has set in.

Another herb is locally called 'The Seven Sisters'. It is called this name, because seven sprouts grow from a long stem. Inside in this stem there is a white milky substance and this is rubbed to warts nine days in succession.

A herb called 'Buglass' is a well known herb in this locality. It has a long stem, large leaves, and a small yellow flower, in the Season of Spring. The leaves are got and warmed near a fire, then broken into small pieces, and put on a sore foot.

> **A very small herb grows on walls or stony parts of fields, and it is locally called 'Saint John'. It is called this name, because it is supposed that Saint John first used this herb as a cure for a sore mouth. It is used still by the people. The herb is boiled, and the juice is rubbed to the sore mouth. (Annie Carroll, Fairfield)**

Sore mouth

The Schools' Collection, Volume 0029, Page 0359

> **A very small herb grows on walls or stony parts of fields, and it is locally called 'Saint John'. It is called this name, because it is supposed that Saint John first used this herb as a cure for a sore mouth. It is used still by the people. The herb is boiled, and the juice is rubbed to the sore mouth.**

This reflects St John's wort's external use as a healing and anti-inflammatory remedy. Priest & Priest described St John's wort as a sedative nervine for muscular twitching and is especially indicated for nerve injuries to the extremities and teeth/gums. St John's wort has been used for facial neuralgia after dental extractions and toothache.

The Egyptian Drug Authority monograph for St John's wort outlines many of the herb's historical uses that have continued into modernity, including skin inflammation, burns and wounds (Egyptian Herbal Monograph, 2022).

St. John's wort's anti-inflammatory, vulnerary, analgesic, astringent, antispasmodic and antimicrobial actions make it a powerful aid for wounds, bruises, burns, sprains and muscle pain and spasms (Hoffmann, 2003; McBride, n.d.; McIntyre, 2019; Smith, 2008; Wood, 1997). Its antiseptic properties help forestall infection in wounds and burns (Chevallier, 1996). Topical applications of an infused oil or salve are commonly used for these purposes.

St John's wort is helpful for neuralgic pain and will ease fibrositis, sciatica and rheumatic pain (Hoffmann, 2003).

St John's wort – other uses

When taken internally, St John's wort is a hugely popular ally that has been used to treat neuralgia, anxiety, stress, and other related issues because of its calming and pain-relieving properties. It is thought to be particularly suitable for use when anxiety and irritability are brought on by menopausal changes.

St John's wort is increasingly recommended to treat depression, an indication that is supported by numerous clinical trials in Europe and the United States.

St John's wort may affect the expression of P-glycoprotein and cytochrome-P (CYP) family enzymes, which are involved in the metabolism of certain medications. This may cause some medications to have altered effects, which could result in less effective outcomes or unanticipated consequences.

Common medications whose effects may be lessened by St John's wort include some oral contraceptive pills, warfarin (an anticoagulant medication), cyclosporin (often used as an immunosuppressant in organ transplants), digoxin (mostly used for atrial fibrillation), proton pump inhibitors (used to reduce stomach acid production), and some statins (drugs that lower cholesterol).

Taking St John's wort with other antidepressants that raise serotonin levels (such as SSRIs and MAOIs) may increase the risk of serotonin syndrome, sometimes referred to as serotonin toxicity, a potentially lethal condition characterised by an excessive build-up of serotonin in the body. The symptoms of serotonin syndrome include sweating, dilated pupils, high blood pressure and elevated body temperatures.

Although St John's wort has been associated with fewer side effects than some antidepressant medications, the most common negative effects associated with its use include gastrointestinal issues and photosensitivity.

St John's wort recipes

St John's wort infused oil

Use this infused oil for painful or sunburned skin.

½ cup fresh St John's wort (*Hypericum perforatum*) aerial parts

2 cups (16 fl oz) olive oil

1. Place fresh St John's wort on a drying screen and let it wilt for at least 24 hours to remove part of the moisture before adding oil.
2. Place wilted plant material in a clean, dry, quart-sized glass canning jar.
3. Cover plant material with room-temperature oil, ensuring that the oil is at least 1 inch above the top of the plants and that the herbs are fully covered.
4. Use a clean, dry spoon to mix thoroughly so that all surfaces of the herb are coated and no air bubbles remain.
5. To shield oil from any chemical coating on the lid, place a square piece of natural waxed paper on top of the jar and cover it with a lid.
6. For 4 to 6 weeks, keep the jar in a warm, dark place. To assist, mix the contents and release the compounds of the herb into the oil by rolling the jar in your palms every 1 to 3 days.
7. Decant the oil after 4–6 weeks. Place a clean, dry, cheesecloth-lined strainer inside a large, clean, dry bowl with a spout. Pour the contents from the jar into the strainer.

8. Pour slowly, paying special attention to any watery layer at the bottom to prevent it from combining with the oil; decant just the oily part and throw away any water or oil that comes into contact with the water. Squeeze the leftover herb oil into the bowl while holding the cheesecloth ends together with clean, dry fingertips.

9. Set aside the leftover herbs for compost.

10. After pouring the oil into a dry, clean jar, cover it and leave it for a few days or overnight.

11. Strain the oil again, being careful to avoid pouring out any of the remaining herb particulates that have settled to the bottom of the jar and avoid pouring out any water layer on the bottom of the jar.

12. Transfer the oil into a clean and dry dark-coloured bottle or jar. Tightly cap.

13. Label and keep for up to a year in a cool, dark place.

Safety considerations

No adverse reactions have been confirmed at dose levels up to 1 mg of total hypericin. Photosensitisation at high doses has been reported during experimental antiviral treatment with synthetic hypericin (35 mg intravenously) in HIV-positive patients. While a few instances of photosensitisation have been documented, this appears to be very rare.

A recent study utilising human keratinocyte cell cultures demonstrated that usual therapeutic doses of *Hypericum* extracts are about 30 to 50 times below the phototoxic level. There have been reports of elevated serotonin levels in patients taking selective serotonin reuptake inhibitors (e.g., sertraline) in combination with St John's wort. Evidence suggests that St John's wort affects the hepatic cytochrome P450 system, increasing the activity of its most abundant isozyme, CYP3A4.

Thus, theoretically, the herb could reduce the activity of simultaneously administered drugs that are known substrates for this isozyme, including non-sedating antihistamines, oral contraceptives, certain antiretroviral agents, antiepileptic medications, calcium channel-blockers, cyclosporine, some chemotherapeutic drugs, macrolide antibiotics and selected antifungals (Hoffmann, 2003).

VIOLET

Viola odorata

The Schools' Collection, Volume 0223, Page 0268

Cures for cramps:
Place a 'man-keeper' on a black sally and bring a branch of the black sally with you, and when the animal is affected rub the branch of the sally to him.
Cure for wild fire:
Write the person's name in ink around the wild fire.
Cure of evil eye cast on cattle:
Write all the letter of the alphabet on a piece of paper and burn it on a plate under the animal's nose. This will break the spell.
To prevent black leg in cattle:
Place a lump of garlic under the skin.
Cure for burn:
Rub a mixture of lime water and linseed oil to it.
Cure of red water in cattle:
Boil rusted iron and give the water as a drink to the cattle.
Cure for jaundice:
Boil wild voilets in milk and drink the milk.

The Schools' Collection, Volume 0500, Page 0074

Burn leaf of cabbage and apply it to sore head and it would cure it.

Boil wild violets and drink the juice and it would cure a pain in the head.

Burn a leaf called hartstongue and apply it to burn and it would cure it.

A cure for a sore throat is to boil the juice of a dandelion and drink the juice.

To rub the milk of a plant called spurge to warts and it would cure them. Tea was made long ago from sloe leaves the method for making the tea was to dry the leaves and put them into teapot and make it the same as ordinary tea. Tea was also made from agrimony,

Got from my mother Michael Hennessy age 54 Ballingarry

The Schools' Collection, Volume 0676, Page 0092

... fresh crops of weeds year after year.

The "Comfry root" is used as a cure for sprains. The "Dandelion" is a cure for warts. The "Garlice" root is used as for runing ear. The wild violet cures broken skin.

The "Comfry root" the "Garlice" and the "wild violet" are applied as a hot poultice to the effected parts. The milk of the Dandelion is rubbed on the warts

One of the herbs used as a food is watercress You can make a food called "angelica" from cow parsley.

Poison is made from "acconite"

The Schools' Collection, Volume 0223, Page 0268

Cure for jaundice:

Boil wild voilets in milk and drink the milk.

The Schools' Collection, Volume 0500, Page 0074

Boil wild violets and drink the juice and it would cure a pain in the head.

The Schools' Collection, Volume 0676, Page 0092

The "Comfry root" is used as a cure for sprains. The "Dandelion" is a cure for warts. The "Garlice" root is used as for runing ear. The wild violet cures broken skin.
The "Comfry root" the "Garlice" and the "wild violet" are applied as a hot poultice to the effected parts. The milk of the Dandelion is rubbed on the warts

A clinical study by Khorsand et al. (2019) evaluated the effects of violet-infused almond oil on pruritus in those undergoing hemodialysis for chronic kidney disease. The study found that violet oil massaged into the skin was more effective for lessening the severity of symptoms than massage alone.

Some herbalists make use of violet's demulcent and diuretic properties to soothe painful, burning urination in cystitis and urinary tract infections (Hardin, n.d.; Hoffmann, 2003). Wood (2008) also lists kidney stones among the many indications of violet.

Violet root is used in remedies for coughs, colds, bronchitis and sore throats because of its expectorant and stimulating effects. The root is also used to make eyewashes and mouthwashes, and to treat thrush. Violet leaf tea can also be drunk for coughs. The leaves are considered to be antiseptic and can be used externally as a compress or taken internally as a tea (Harford, 2019).

Violet recipes

Lymphatic massage oil

2 parts violet (*Viola* spp.) aerial parts infused oil

2 parts calendula (*Calendula officinalis*) flower infused oil

1 drop of vitamin E oil (optional)

1. See "How to make a herbal infused oil" (page 46).

2. Measure the appropriate amount of each herbal oil and transfer to a dark-coloured, sanitised, dry glass container.

3. Add vitamin E oil, if using.

4. Cover and shake well to combine.

5. Label, and store in a cool, dark place for up to 1 year.

Spring facial steam

¼ cup calendula (*Calendula officinalis*) flowers

¼ cup chamomile (*Matricaria chamomilla*) flowers

⅛ cup lavender (*Lavandula* spp.) flower buds

⅛ cup nettle (*Urtica dioica*) leaf

⅛ cup red clover (*Trifolium pratense*) flowers

⅛ cup violet (*Viola* spp.) flowers

1. Combine all herbs together and mix well. Place mixture in a labelled, air-tight, dry glass jar and store in a cool, dark location such as a cupboard.

2. Bring a pot of water (about 4 quarts) to a boil, then carefully pour hot water into a large, heat-safe bowl (glass, ceramic or stainless steel).

3. Add ½ cup of the herb mixture to the bowl and stir briefly with a spoon.

4. Sit with your face at a comfortable distance (approximately 6–12 inches) above the bowl, and cover your head and the bowl with a towel or blanket to capture the steam.

5. Steam your skin for about 5–10 minutes, then quickly rinse with cool water to tighten pores.

Violet vinegar

½ cup violet (*Viola* spp.) flowers

1½ cups white wine vinegar

1. Gather your violet flowers.
2. Rinse them thoroughly with cool water and let dry.
3. Place violets in a pint-sized glass jar and pour vinegar over the top. If you are using a metal lid, place parchment paper over the jar's top before closing it.
4. Allow the violets to infuse in the vinegar overnight or until the infusion turns beautifully pink.
5. Strain the violets.

Violet vinaigrette

1 cup extra virgin olive oil

¼ cup violet vinegar

¼ tsp garlic powder

1 tbsp minced wild onions (*Allium* spp.) (optional)

1 tsp local honey

½ tsp ground Himalayan sea salt

¼ tsp black pepper

1. Combine all ingredients in a glass jar and shake until the vinaigrette is combined.
2. Use immediately on fresh salad or foraged greens.
3. Store in the glass jar in the refrigerator for 3–5 days.

Safety considerations

Some people are sensitive to violets and may experience a slight burning sensation in the throat after consumption, particularly with the raw plant (Bergo, n.d.).

YARROW

Achillea millefolium

The Schools' Collection, Volume 0043, Page 0032

Local Cures:

1. Gosthune

An herb. It cures boils. It looks like a nettle. Grows about 2 feet high. The leaf is warmed and applied to the boil.

2. Yarrow

Is used for rheumatism. A green herb with a white top. It grows to a height of about six inches. It is stewed in hot water for about five minutes. It is cooled and then drunk.

The Schools' Collection, Volume 0043, Page 0045

The yarrow is a small stalk with a white top on it. It is used for curing rheumatism by stewing it in hot water for about five hours. It is taken up then and the juice put in a bottle to cool and it is then drunk.

The Schools' Collection, Volume 0047, Page 0068

Yarrow is a plant which grows on the road-side near Newtown or in Mr. Barry's land. The flower is of a reddish colour with grey spots. This is cut off the stem and chopped up and boiled until it becomes quite soft. Then it is mixed with the juice of a carrot and the old people used it as a cure for sciatica.

Rheumatism

The Schools' Collection, Volume 0043, Page 0032

Yarrow.
Is used for rheumatism. A green herb with a white top. It grows to a height of about six inches. It is stewed in hot water for about five minutes. It is cooled and then drunk.

The Schools' Collection, Volume 0043, Page 0045

The yarrow is a small stalk with a white top on it. It is used for curing rheumatism by stewing it in hot water for about five hours. It is taken up then and the juice put in a bottle to cool and it is then drunk.

In Ireland, there has been a tradition among older people of drinking yarrow tea in the belief that it combats rheumatism and the pain of arthritis. It has since been discovered that yarrow contains a salt, phosphate of soda, which is lacking in those who suffer from this complaint.

To prepare yarrow, gather the blossoms just before they begin to flower. Dry the leaves/flowers gently and quickly at room temperature. Add 1 oz of the herb to 1 pint of boiling water to infuse. Leave in a covered jug for about 10 minutes and take half a cup 3 times per day between meals or before eating.

Similar uses of yarrow are seen in the Persian traditions, where it is used to support wound health, pneumonia, rheumatism and blood loss (Saeidnia et al., 2011).

Yarrow is an excellent diaphoretic, often used in teas to promote sweating, thereby helping reduce fevers. Yarrow is a classic first-aid herb and can be used to stop bleeding both internally and externally. It is effective for both menstrual and stomach cramps and is often used in formulas for stomach flu. It also has beneficial effects for the heart and lungs (Gladstar, 2012).

Hool (1922) notes that owing to its diuretic and alterative properties, yarrow can also be an appropriate herb for dissolving uric acid crystals and other hard calculus deposits. This also makes yarrow a beneficial plant for addressing arthritic conditions, including gout and rheumatism. It can be combined with buchu (*Agathosma betulina*) leaf, goldenrod (*Solidago* spp.) aerial parts, pellitory of the wall (*Parietaria judaica*) aerial parts, sea holly (*Eryngium maritimum*) root, and / or uva ursi (*Arctostaphylos uva-ursi*) leaf in formulations for these concerns (Hool, 1922).

Yarrow is a urinary antiseptic and has been used for infections such as cystitis. Used externally, it will aid in the healing of wounds. Yarrow is used for a wide variety of common acute complaints including the treatment of common cold, flu, fevers, hypertension, painful menstruation and bleeding.

Yarrow is styptic. It is often mixed with shepherd's purse, another powerful styptic, as first aid to staunch excessive bleeding, whether from a cut, a deep wound or a simple nosebleed. For this reason, Yarrow and Shepherd's purse is a very popular remedy for menorraghia often combined with nettle due to nettle's fantastic nutritive and tonic qualities.

Yarrow has been used with elder flowers, peppermint, boneset, cayenne and ginger for fevers. Yarrow also has antispasmodic properties and is used to relieve both menstrual and stomach cramps. It is often combined with ginger for this purpose, whether taken internally or applied topically as a poultice (Gladstar, 2012).

Sciatica

The Schools' Collection, Volume 0047, Page 0068

Yarrow is a plant which grows on the road-side near Newtown or in Mr. Barry's land The flower is of a reddish colour with grey

> **spots. This is cut off the stem and chopped up and boiled until it becomes quite soft. Then it is mixed with the juice of a carrot and the old people used it as a cure for sciatica.**

The Thompson Native Americans also boiled yarrow roots and leaves for bathing arthritic limbs. The roots were pounded and used as a poultice on the skin for sciatica (Turner et al., 1990).

Yarrow recipes

First sign of illness tea

3g (0.1 oz) elder (*Sambucus nigra* or *S. canadensis*) flower

3g (0.1 oz) yarrow (*Achillea millefolium*) aerial parts

3g (0.1 oz) peppermint (*Mentha x piperita*) leaf

1. Pour 475 ml (16 fl oz) hot water over 9g (0.3 oz) tea blend.
2. Let steep for 10–15 minutes, covered.
3. Strain and drink while hot.
4. Keep the body and feet insulated and warm for 1 hour after drinking this tea.

Heavy bleed menstrual / menopause tea

Have a week before your bleed as a tea and then while bleeding.

Yarrow (*Achillea millefolium*) aerial parts

Shepherd's purse (*Capsella bursa-pastoris*) aerial parts

Nettle (*Urtica dioica*) leaf

1. Mix equal parts of each herb.

2. Place your herbs directly into your cafetière or infuser. Pour hot water over herbs.
3. Cover the mug or teapot immediately with a lid or saucer. This traps the steam and prevents the medicinal essential oils from evaporating.
4. Let the mixture steep undisturbed for 10 to 15 minutes.
5. Remove the infuser or strain the liquid into your cup. Drink it plain, or add honey and lemon to taste.

Soothing skin oil

3 parts calendula (*Calendula officinalis*) flower infused oil

3 parts lavender (*Lavandula spp.*) flower bud infused oil

3 parts yarrow (*Achillea millefolium*) aerial parts infused oil

1. See "How to make a herbal infused oil" (page 46).
2. Measure the appropriate amount of each herbal oil and transfer to a dark-coloured, sanitised, dry glass container. Cover and shake well to combine.
3. Label, and store in a cool, dark place for up to 1 year.

Safety considerations

Hypersensitivity to yarrow and other plants in the Asteraceae family has been reported. Some authorities caution against using *Achillea* during pregnancy. No restrictions during lactation are suggested (Hoffmann, 2003).

BIBLIOGRAPHY

Almqvist, B. (1977–79). "The Irish Folklore Commission: Achievement and Legacy". Béaloideas 45/47: 6–26. doi:10.2307/ 20521388. JSTOR 20521388.

American Botanical Council. (1999). The Complete German Commission E Monographs: Elecampane. Available at http://cms.herbalgram.org/commissione/Monographs/Monograph0091.html (Accessed: 18 February 2026).

Angier, B. (2008). Field Guide to Medicinal Wild Plants. 2nd edn. Mechanicsburg, PA: Stackpole Books.

Barna, M., Kucera, A., Hladikova, M. and Kucera, M. (2012). Randomized double-blind study: Wound-healing effects of a *Symphytum* herb extract cream (*Symphytum* × *uplandicum* Nyman) in children. *Arzneimittel-Forschung*, 62(6): 285–289.

Bennett, R.R. (2014). *The Gift of Healing Herbs*. Berkeley, CA: North Atlantic Books.

Bergo, A. (n.d.). Violets. Retrieved from https://foragerchef.com/violets/

Blair, K. (2014). *The Wild Wisdom of Weeds: 13 Essential Plants for Human Survival*. White River Junction, VT: Chelsea Green Publishing.

Blumenthal, M. (1998). *The Complete German Commission E Monographs: Therapeutic Guide to Herbal Medicine*. Boston, MA: American Botanical Council.

Bone, K. and Mills, S. (2013). *Principles and Practice of Phytotherapy: Modern Herbal Medicine*. 2nd edn. Edinburgh: Churchill Livingstone.

Bordia, A., Verma, S.K. and Srivastava, K.C. (1998). Effect of garlic (*Allium sativum*) on blood lipids, blood sugar, fibrinogen and fibrinolytic activity in patients with coronary artery disease. *Prostaglandins Leukot Essential Fatty Acids*, 58(4): 257–263.

Boughman, A.L. and Oxendine, L.O. (2003). *Herbal Remedies of the Lumbee Indians*. Jefferson, NC: McFarland & Company.

Briody, M. (2007). *The Irish Folklore Commission, 1935–1970: History, Ideology, Methodology*. Helsinki: Finnish Literature Society

Brown, T. (1985). *Tom Brown's Field Guide: Wild Edible and Medicinal Plants*. New York: Berkley Books.

Bruton-Seal, J. and Seal, Matthew. (2008). *Hedgerow Medicine: Harvest and Make Your Own Herbal Remedies*. Ludlow, UK: Merlin Unwin Books.

Budoff, M. (2006). Aged garlic extract retards progression of coronary artery calcification. *The Journal of Nutrition*, 136(3): 741S–744S.

Cech, R. (2000). *Making Plant Medicine*. Williams, OR: Horizon Herbs.

Cech, R. (2016). *Making Plant Medicine*. 4th edn. Herbal Reads LLC.

Chandler, R.F., Freeman, L. and Hooper, S.N. (1979). Herbal remedies of the Maritime Indians. *Journal of Ethnopharmacology*, 1(1): 49–68.

Charousaei, F., Dabirian, A. and Mojab, F. (2011). Using chamomile solution or a 1% topical hydrocortisone ointment in the management of peristomal skin lesions in colostomy patients: Results of a controlled clinical study. *Ostomy/Wound Management*, 57(5): 28–36.

Chevallier, A. (1996). *The Encyclopedia of Medicinal Plants*. New York: DK Publishing, Inc.

Chevallier, A. (2007). *Herbal Remedies*. New York: DK Publishing.

Cook, W.H. (1869). *The Physiomedical Dispensatory: A Treatise on Therapeutics, Materia Medica, and Pharmacy*. Cincinnati. OH: Published by the author.

Culpeper, N. (1995). *Culpeper's Complete Herbal: A Book of Natural Remedies for Ancient Ills*. Ware, UK: Wordsworth Editions. (Original work published 1653.)

de Souza, M.M., de Jesus, R.A.P., Cechinel-Filho, V. and Schlemper, V. (1998). Analgesic profile of hydroalcoholic extract obtained from *Marrubium vulgare*. *Phytomedicine*, 5(2): 103–107.

Dioscorides. (2000). *De Materia Medica*. Translated by T.E. Osbaldeston. Johannesburg, South Africa: Ibidis Press. (Original work published 70 CE.)

Easley, T. and Horne, S. (2016). *The Modern Herbal Dispensary: A Medicine-making Guide*. Berkeley, CA: North Atlantic Books.

Edwards, G.F. (2000). *Opening Our Wild Hearts to the Healing Herbs*. Woodstock, NY: Ash Tree Publishing.

Egyptian Herbal Monograph. (2022). *Hypericum perforatum*, pp. 301–307. Egyptian Drug Authority.

El Bardai, S., Morel, N., Wibo, M., Fabre, N., Llabres, G., Lyoussi, B. and Quetin-Leclercq, J. (2003). The vasorelaxant activity of marrubenol and marrubiin from *Marrubium vulgare*. *Planta Medica*, 69(1): 75–77.

El Bardai, S., Lyoussi, B., Wibo, M. and Morel, N. (2004). Comparative study of the antihypertensive activity of *Marrubium vulgare* and of the dihydropyridine calcium antagonist amlodipine in spontaneously hypertensive rat. *Clinical and Experimental Hypertension*, 26(6): 465–474.

Ellingwood, F. (1919). *The American Materia Medica, Therapeutics and Pharmacognosy*. Evanston, IL: Ellingwood's Therapeutist.

European Medicines Agency. (2015). *European Union Herbal Monograph on Matricaria recutita L., flos*. Available at: https://www.ema.europa.eu (Accessed: 18 February 2026).

Felter, H.W. (1922). *The Eclectic Materia Medica, Pharmacology, and Therapeutics*. Cincinnati, OH: Scudder, J.K.

Foster, S. (1993). *Herbal Renaissance*. Layton, UT: Peregrine Smith Books.

Foster, S. (2009). *Milk Thistle Monograph*. Stephen Foster Group, Inc.

Gardner, Z. and McGuffin, M. (2013). *American Herbal Products Association's Botanical Safety Handbook*. Boca Raton, FL: CRC Press.

Garran, T.A. (2008). *Western Herbs According to Traditional Chinese Medicine*. Rochester, VT: Healing Arts Press.

Garrett, J.T. (2003). *The Cherokee Herbal: Native Plant Medicine from the Four Directions*. Rochester, VT: Bear & Company.

Gladstar, R. (1993). *Herbal Healing for Women*. New York: Simon & Schuster.

Gladstar, R. (2001). *Herbal Recipes for Vibrant Health.* Adams, MA: Storey Publishing.

Gladstar, R. (2012). *The Science and Art of Herbalism.* Online course. https://scienceandartofherbalism.com/

Grieve, M. (1971). *A Modern Herbal.* Vols 1 & 2. New York: Dover Publications. (Original work published 1931.)

Haas, E. (2006). *Staying Healthy with Nutrition.* New York: Ten Speed Press.

Hall, D. (1988). *Creating Your Herbal Profile.* New Canaan, CT: Keats Publishing.

Hamel, P.B. and Chiltoskey, M.U. (1975). *Cherokee Plants and Their Uses: A 400 Year History.* Sylva, NC: Herald Publishing Co.

Hardin, K.R. (n.d.). *Three Faces under a Hood: The Many Aspects of Violet.* Available at: https://enchantersgreen.com/violet (Accessed: 18 February 2026).

Harford, R. (2019). *Edible and Medicinal Wild Plants of Britain and Ireland.* Self-published.

Heckels, F., Lawton, K. and Benfield, B. (2019). *The Sensory Herbal Handbook: Connect with the Medicinal Power of Your Local Plants.* London: Watkins Publishing.

Helms, S. and Miller, A. (2006). Natural treatment of chronic rhinosinusitis. *Alternative Medicine Review,* 11(3): 196–207.

Hoffelt, S. (2016). Yellow dock's versatile history. *Natural Herbal Living,* March, pp. 19–25.

Hoffmann, D. (1988). *The Herbal Handbook.* Rochester, VT: Healing Arts Press.

Hoffmann, D. (1993). *An Elders' Herbal.* Rochester, VT: Healing Art Press.

Hoffmann, D. (2003). *Medical Herbalism: The Science and Practice of Herbal Medicine*. Rochester, VT: Healing Arts Press.

Hoffmann, D. (no date). *Is Comfrey Safe?* Available at: http://www.herbcraft.org/hoffmanncomfrey.html (Accessed: 18 February 2026).

Holmes, P. (1989). *The Energetics of Western Herbs*. Vol 1. Boulder, CO: Snow Lotus Press.

Hool, R.L. (1922). *Common Plants and Their Uses in Medicine: Containing Explanatory Articles on the Treatment of Disease with Non-poisonous Herbal Remedies, also Short Biographical Notes*. Bolton: Lancashire Branch of the National Association of Medical Herbalists.

Horton, J., Goldstein, J. and Brown, M. (2002). SREBPs: Activators of the complete program of cholesterol and fatty acid synthesis in the liver. *Journal of Clinical Investigation*, 109(9): 1125–1131.

Hussain, K., Zia-ul-Hussnain, S. and Shahazas, A. (2010). Distributions and folk Tibb knowledge of milk thistle (*Silybum marianum* L.) in NWFP, Pakistan. *Ethnobotanical Leaflets*, 14: 268–273.

Kanak, S., Krzemińska, B., Berecka-Rycerz, A., Kopeć, M. and Dos Santos Szewczyk, K. (2025). Harnessing the power of *Alchemilla*: A natural solution for skin health and dermatological disorders. *Molecules*, 30(8): 1861.

Katz, S. (2000). Eyebright. In Gladstar, R. and Hirsch, P. (eds.) *Planting the Future: Saving Our Medicinal Herbs*. Rochester, VT: Healing Arts Press, pp. 100–104.

Katz, N.J. (2016). Yellow dock herbal monograph. *Natural Herbal Living*, March, pp. 4–9.

Khorsand, A., Salari, R., Noras, M.R., Saki, A., Jamali, J., Sharifipour, F. and Ghazanfari, S.M. (2019). The effect of massage and topical violet oil on the severity of pruritus and dry skin in hemodialysis patients: randomized controlled trial. *Complementary Therapies in Medicine*, 45: 248–253.

Kianbakht, S., Khalighi-Sigaroodi, F. and Dabaghian, F.H. (2013). Improved glycemic control in patients with advanced type 2 diabetes mellitus taking *Urtica dioica* leaf extract. *Clinical Laboratory*, 59(9–10): 1071–1076.

Kianitalaei, A., Feyzabadi, Z., Hamedi, S. and Qaraaty, M. (2019). *Althaea officinalis* in traditional medicine and modern phytotherapy. *Journal of Advanced Pharmacy Education & Research*, 9(S2): 154–161.

Klenner, A. (2016). Smooth digestion through yellow dock. *Natural Herbal Living*, March, pp. 27–32.

Klenner, A., Holfelt, S., Nunez, M., Katz, N., Morgan, J. and Little, C. (2015). Chickweed. *Natural Herbal Living Magazine*, Issue 19.

Kress, H. (2004). *Nettle Seed*. Available at: https://www.henriettes-herb.com/blog/nettle-seed.html (Accessed: 18 February 2026).

Kuhn, M. and Winston, D. (2008). *Herbal Therapy & Supplements*. 2nd edn. Philadelphia, PA: Lippincott Williams & Wilkins.

Lloyd, J.U. and Felter, H.W. (1898). *King's American Dispensatory*. 18th edn. Cincinnati, OH: Ohio Valley Co.

Luchterhand, C. (2012). *Gastroesophageal Reflux Disease (GERD) Patient Handout*. University of Wisconsin-Madison School of Medicine and Public Health.

Lyle, T.J. (1897). *Physio-Medical Therapeutics, Materia Medica and Pharmacology*. The National Association of Medical Herbalists of Great Britain.

Masé, G. (2013). *The Wild Medicine Solution: Healing with Aromatic, Bitter, and Tonic Plants*. Rochester, VT: Healing Arts Press.

McBride, K. (no date). *5 Healing Uses of St. John's Wort Oil*. Available at: https://kamimcbride.com (Accessed: 18 February 2026).

McIntyre, A. (1996). *Flower Power*. New York: Henry Holt and Company, Inc.

McIntyre, A. (2019). *The Complete Herbal Tutor: The Definitive Guide to the Principles and Practices of Herbal Medicine*. 2nd edn. London: Aeon Books.

McIntyre, A. (no date). *Milk Thistle: Silybum marianum (Monograph)*. Available at: http://annemcintyre.com (Accessed: 18 February 2026).

Mei, N., Guo, L., Fu, P.P., Heflich, R.H. and Chen, T. (2005). Mutagenicity of comfrey (*Symphytum officinale*) in rat liver. *British Journal of Cancer*, 92(5): 873–875.

Merfort, I., Heilmann, J., Hagedorn-Leweke, U. and Lippold, B.C. (1994). In vivo skin penetration studies of camomile flavones. *Die Pharmazie*, 49(7): 509–511.

Mittman, P. (1990). Randomized, double-blind study of freeze-dried *Urtica dioica* in the treatment of allergic rhinitis. *Planta Medica*, 56(1): 44–47.

Moerman, D. (2009). *Native American Medicinal Plants*. Portland, OR: Timber Press.

Moore, M. (2003). *Medicinal Plants of the Mountain West*. Santa Fe, NM: Museum of New Mexico Press.

Native American Ethnobotany Database. (2003). *Petroselinum crispum* [Online database]. Retrieved from http://naeb.brit.org/uses/search/?string=Petroselinum+crispum

NIH (National Institute of Health). (2019). "Zinc Fact Sheet". Retrieved 23 May 2019, from https://ods.od.nih.gov/factsheets/Zinc-HealthProfessional/

Nowak, A., Klimowicz, A., Bielecka-Grzela, S. and Piechota, M. (2012). Inulin: A valuable nutritional component. *Annales Academiae Medicae Stetinensis*, 58(1): 62–65.

Ody, P. (2017). *The Complete Medicinal Herbal*. New York: Skyhorse Publishing.

Orekhov, A.N. and Grunwald, J. (1997). Effects of garlic on atherosclerosis. *Nutrition*, 13(7): 656–663.

Paine, A. (2006). *The Healing Power of Celtic Plants*. Washington, USA: John Hunt Publishing.

Pedersen, M. (1998). *Nutritional Herbology*. Whitman Publications.

Pengelly, A. (2004). *The Constituents of Medicinal Plants*. 2nd edn. Cambridge, MA: CABI Publishing.

Potterton, D. (Ed.). (2002). *Culpeper's Color Herbal*. New York: Sterling Publishing.

Priest, A.W. & Priest, L.R. (1982). *Herbal Medication – A Clinical and Dispensary Handbook*. Romford, Essex: L.N. Fowler & Co.

Rahimi-Madiseh, M., Lorigoini, Z., Zamani-Gharaghoshi, H. and Rafieian-Kopaei, M. (2017). *Berberis vulgaris*: Specifications and traditional uses. *Iranian Journal of Basic Medical Sciences, 20*(5): 569. http://doi.org/10.22038/IJBM S.2017.8690

Randall, C., Randall, H., Dobbs, F., Hutton, C. and Sanders, H. (2000). Randomized controlled trial of nettle sting for treatment of base-of-thumb pain. *Journal of the Royal Society of Medicine, 93*(6): 305–309. https://doi.org/10.1177/014107680009300607

Rayburn, K., Fleischbein, E., Song, J., Allen, B., Kundert, M., Leiter, C. and Bush, T. (2009). Stinging nettle cream for osteoarthritis. *Alternative Therapies in Health and Medicine, 15*(4): 60–61.

Reinhart, K.M. (2008). Effects of garlic on blood pressure in patients with and without systolic hypertension: A meta-analysis. *Annals of Pharmacotherapy*, 42(12): 1766–1771.

Romm, A. (2024). *Natural Medicine Chest for Kids' Immunity*. Available at: https://avivaromm.com (Accessed: 18 February 2026).

Rose, J. (1972). *Herbs & Things*. New York: Grosset & Dunlap.

Saeidnia, S., Gohari, A., Mokhber-Dezfuli, N. and Kiuchi, F. (2011). A review on phytochemistry and medicinal properties of the genus *Achillea*. *DARU Journal of Pharmaceutical Sciences,* 19(3), 173–186. https://www.ncbi.nlm.nih.gov/pmc/articles/PMC3232110/#CIT0011

Safarinejad, M.R. (2005). *Urtica dioica* for treatment of benign prostatic hyperplasia: A prospective, randomized, double-blind, placebo-controlled, crossover study. *Journal of Herbal Pharmacotherapy,* 5(4): 1–11.

Salmón, E. (2020). *Iwígara: The Kinship of Plants and People: American Indian Ethnobotanical Traditions and Science.* Portland, OR: Timber Press, Inc.

Scallan, C. (1994). *Irish Herbal Cures*. Dublin: Gill & Macmillan.

Scott, M. ed. (1986). *An Irish Herbal: The Botanologia Universalis Hibernica of John K'eogh*. Wellingborough: Aquarian Press.

Silagy, C.A., Neil, W. and Andrew, H. (1994). A meta-analysis of the effect of garlic on blood pressure. *Journal of Hypertension*, 12(4): 463–468.

Skenderi, G. (2003). *Herbal Vade Mecum*. Rutherford, NJ: Herbacy Press.

Smith, E. (2008). *Therapeutic Herb Manual: A Guide to the Safe and Effective Use of Liquid Herbal Extracts*. Self-published.

Srivastava, J.K., Shankar, E. and Gupta, S. (2010). Chamomile: A herbal medicine of the past with a bright future. *Molecular Medicine Reports*, 3(6): 895–901.

Stevinson, C., Pittler, M.H. and Ernst, E. (2000). Garlic for treating hypercholesterolemia: A meta-analysis of randomized clinical trials. *Annals of Internal Medicine*, 133(6): 420–429.

Storl, W.D. (2012). *The Herbal Lore of Wise Women and Wortcunners*. Berkeley, CA: North Atlantic Books.

Tasić-Kostov, M., Arsić, I., Pavlović, D., Stojanović, S., Najman, S., Naumović, S. and Tadić, V. (2019). Towards a modern approach to traditional use: In vitro and in vivo evaluation of *Alchemilla vulgaris* L. gel wound healing potential. *Journal of Ethnopharmacology*, 238: 111789.

Tierra, M. (1988). *Planetary Herbology*. Twin Lakes, WI: Lotus Press.

Tierra, M. (1998). *The Way of Chinese Herbs*. New York: Simon & Schuster Inc.

Tierra, L. (2003). *Healing with the Herbs of Life*. Berkeley, CA: Ten Speed Press.

Tilgner, S. (2009). *Herbal Medicine from the Heart of the Earth*. Pleasant Hills, OR: Wise Acres LLC.

Tillotson, A.K. (2001). *The One Earth Herbal Sourcebook*. New York: Kensington Publishing Group.

Turner, N.J., Thompson, L.C., Thompson, M.T. and York, A.Z. (1990). Thompson Ethnobotany: Knowledge and Usage of Plants by the Thompson Indians of British Columbia. Victoria: Royal British Columbia Museum.

Van Wyk, B-E. and Wink, M. (2014). *Phytomedicines, Herbal Drugs, and Poisons*. London: Kew Publishing.

Whelan, R. (no date). *Marshmallow*. Available at: http://www.rjwhelan.co.nz/herbs%20A-Z/marshmallow.html (Accessed: 18 February 2026).

Winston, D. and Maimes, S. (2019). *Adaptogens: Herbs for Strength, Stamina, and Stress Relief*. 2nd edn. Rochester, VT: Healing Arts Press.

Wood, C. (2009). *Chickweed: My Favourite Salad Green*. Available at: http://www.susunweed.com/herbal_ezine/February09/grandmother.htm (Accessed: 18 February 2026).

Wood, M. (1997). *The Book of Herbal Wisdom: Using Plants as Medicines*. Berkeley, CA: North Atlantic Books.

Wood, M. (2004) *The Practice of Traditional Western Herbalism: Basic Doctrine, Energetics, and Classification*. Berkeley, CA: North Atlantic Books.

Wood, M. (2008). *The Earthwise Herbal: A Complete Guide to Old World Medicinal Plants*. Berkeley, CA: North Atlantic Books.Young, D., Rogers, R. and Willier, R. (2015). *A Cree Healer and His Medicine Bundle*. Berkeley, CA: North Atlantic Books.

Zarai, Z., Kadri, A., Chobba, I.B., Mansour, R.B., Bekir, A., Mejdoub, H. and Gharsallah, N. (2011). The in-vitro evaluation of antibacterial, antifungal and cytotoxic properties of *Marrubium vulgare* L. essential oil grown in Tunisia. *Lipids in Health and Disease,* 10: 161.

INDEX

www.ingramcontent.com/pod-product-compliance
Lightning Source LLC
LaVergne TN
LVHW011241220926
848584LV00004B/23